MANAGED CARE IN MEDICAID

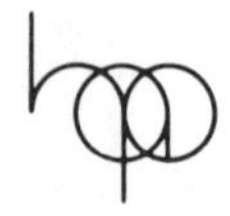

Health Administration Press is a division of the Foundation of the American College of Healthcare Executives. The Editorial Board is a cooperative activity of the Association for Health Services Research and the Foundation of the American College of Healthcare Executives. The Press was established in 1972 with the support of the W. K. Kellogg Foundation.

MANAGED CARE IN MEDICAID

Lessons for Policy and Program Design

Robert E. Hurley
Deborah A. Freund
John E. Paul

Foreword by
Gail R. Wilensky and Louis F. Rossiter

Health Administration Press
Ann Arbor, Michigan 1993

97 96 95 94 93 5 4 3 2 1

Library of Congress Cataloging-in-Publication Data

Hurley, Robert E.
Managed care in Medicaid : lessons for policy and program design / Robert E. Hurley, Deborah A. Freund, John E. Paul.
p. cm.
Includes bibliographical references and index.
ISBN 0-910701-95-4 (softbound : alk. paper)
1. Medicaid. 2. Managed care plans (Medical care)—United States. 3. Insurance, Health—Government policy—United States. I. Freund, Deborah A. II. Paul, John E., date. III. Title.
[DNLM: 1. Managed Care Programs—United States. 2. Medicaid. 3. Primary Health Care—organization & administration. W 275 AA1 H9m 1993]
HD7102.U4H87 1993 368.4'2'00973—dc20
DNLM/DLC for Library of Congress 92-48437 CIP

The paper used in this publication meets the minimum requirements of American National Standard for Information Sciences—Permanence of Paper for Printed Library Materials, ANSI Z39.48-1984. ♾ ™

Health Administration Press
A division of the Foundation of the American College of Healthcare Executives
1021 East Huron Street
Ann Arbor, Michigan 48104-9990
(313) 764-1380

The Association for Health Services Research
1350 Connecticut Avenue, NW
Suite 1100
Washington, DC 20036
(202) 223-2477

The authors gratefully dedicate this book to their understanding and long-suffering spouses—Jenny, Tom, and Jill. The authors also offer a special dedication to the memory of a friend, colleague, and source of much knowledge and many insights, Jean G. Yates.

Contents

List of Abbreviations

AFDC	Aid to Families with Dependent Children
AHCCCS	Arizona Health Care Cost Containment System
AHCPR	Agency for Health Care Policy and Research
ALOS	Average length of stay
BC/BS	Blue Cross/Blue Shield
CMP	Children's Medicaid Program, Suffolk County, State of New York
COBRA	Consolidated Omnibus Budget Reconciliation Act of 1985
CP	Clinic Plan (Michigan)
C/THP	Child/Teen Health Program (New York)
DAHP	Dayton (Ohio) Area Health Plan
DPW	Department of Public Welfare
DRG	Diagnosis-related group
FFS	Fee-for-service
GA	General Assistance
GHAA	Group Health Association of America
GHC	Group Health Cooperative, State of Washington
GOM	Grade of membership
HCFA	Health Care Financing Administration
HIO	Health insuring organization
HMA	Health Management Associates
HMO	Health maintenance organization
HPSM	Health Plan of San Mateo, California
IPA	Independent practice association
KenPAC	Kentucky Patient Access and Care system
KPS	Kitsap Physician Services, Kitsap County, State of Washington
LOS	Length of stay

MA	Medical Assistance (Pennsylvania)
MCD	Medicaid Competition Demonstration
MIS	Management information system
MITS	Multiple interrupted time series
MMIS	Medicaid management information system
MP	Medicaid Personal Physician (New Jersey)
MPE	Medicaid Program Evaluation
MSIS	Medicaid Statistical Information System
NCHSR	National Center for Health Services Research (now AHCPR)
NGA	National Governors' Association
OB-GYN	Obstetrician-gynecologist
OBRA	Omnibus Budget Reconciliation Act of 1981
OLS	Ordinary least squares
ORD	Office of Research and Demonstrations, HCFA
PCCM	Primary care case management
PCM	Primary care manager
PCMP-1	Physician Case Management Program 1 (Children), State of New York
PCN	Primary Care Network (Kansas)
PCP	Primary care physician
PCPP	Primary Care Physician Program (Colorado)
PHP	Prepaid health plan
POD	Pool of doctors (State of Washington)
PPO	Preferred provider organization
PRO	Professional review organization
PSP	Physician Sponsor Plan (Michigan) and Physician Sponsors Plan (Missouri)
RBRVS	Resource-based relative value scale
RTI	Research Triangle Institute
SSI	Supplemental Security Income
UNLV	University of Nevada, Las Vegas
UNR	University of Nevada, Reno
UPA	University Pediatric Associates, State of New York

Foreword

One of the original goals of the Medicaid program was to purchase care in such a way as to avoid the development of a separate, parallel medical benefits program for low-income persons. Medicaid was modeled on traditional Blue Cross/Blue Shield service benefits insurance, to mimic the private sector. Few observers would argue today that this goal has been met. But new and significant opportunities have arisen to move Medicaid beneficiaries into arrangements that are similar or identical to those in the private sector. Alternative financing and delivery systems, subsumed under the rubric of managed or coordinated care systems, have recently seen their Medicaid enrollments grow more rapidly than their private membership. In the past two years, as the direct result of federal policy efforts, Medicaid coordinated care has grown by nearly 50 percent to 3.6 million enrollees. Most states have major new managed care initiatives under way to bring their entire Medicaid enrollment into coordinated care.

While the long-term fate of the Medicaid program may be uncertain, because of both escalating costs and disillusionment over the failings of this program for poor people, discussions about medical assistance to low-income people will continue. As managed care and managed competition become the apparent direction for policy development, the experience to date with managed care in Medicaid will become all the more important. A major policy priority should be the enrollment of as many persons as possible in competitive, network-based health plans through existing sources of coverage. This would push public and private sponsors of coverage to intensify their efforts to engage or build networks of providers who are willing to assume risk and responsibility for serving their enrollees. Moreover, it is likely that some of the successful Medicaid managed care programs will become the foundation for state-sponsored programs for persons who will not be covered by private employers. A number of states, notably Washington, Florida, and New York, are already testing such approaches.

The flexibility that has characterized the Medicaid program in the area of managed care may appear more like confusion to some. But Medicaid has been a wellspring of innovations that few would have predicted just ten years ago. We believe the die is cast and that there is likely to be little slackening in the pace of converting Medicaid programs to coordinated care delivery systems. The conversion will continue to be uneven among the states and will reflect the great diversity in state Medicaid programs and local medical markets.

By the same token, all Medicaid eligibles will not be enrolled in fully integrated systems such as HMOs because these models will not be available everywhere. Other alternatives, such as primary care case management, can offer flexibility, reflecting local provider and consumer preferences in many markets. The special problems of low-income persons, residing mainly in inner-city settings and often with physical or social disabilities, demand delivery systems that are customized to their needs. Thus, the need is not so much for complete mainstream health care for Medicaid beneficiaries as it is for *resemblance* to mainstream systems.

Into this arena enters this volume, the first book-length treatment of Medicaid managed care. Fortunately for us, the readers, the authors have played a substantial role in building the body of knowledge that they attempt to sort out. They do a thorough and rigorous job of sifting through the diversity of more than 25 different initiatives to accomplish two goals: first, to develop a way to organize the evidence to permit legitimate cross-program comparisons; and second, to make those comparisons based on the availability and validity of program findings. They are particularly successful in meeting the first goal of developing an approach to classify the programs and detail similarities and differences in ways meaningful to policymakers, managers, and researchers, who traditionally find it very difficult to communicate about programs with so many different manifestations.

The goal of making comparisons of program impacts on cost and use is more critical and also more complex. The quality of available evidence is mixed and uneven, as the authors describe in detail. The states have experimented at different periods of time, thus background conditions have not been the same and comparisons are difficult. Major technical problems, such as the lack of data from prepaid providers, have not been satisfactorily resolved to permit rigorous analysis. Finally, the programs have often been evaluated in their early stages. Sometimes we need longer periods to see how impacts play out as programs mature. But the authors succeed in presenting a highly informative picture of the Medicaid managed care experience in cost and use. And to their credit, they are modest in drawing their conclusions and frank about the limitations of the growing body of knowledge.

This book, like most sound research, is a source of many answers and many more questions. The reader will be well served to recognize that the decade of program expansion described in this book could be a precursor for another decade of much larger and more inclusive, publicly sponsored managed care initiatives. This new wave of experience with coordinated care and managed competition is likely to draw heavily on the important body of knowledge contained in this volume.

Gail R. Wilensky, Ph.D.
Louis F. Rossiter, Ph.D.

Acknowledgments

The research for this book was sponsored in part by Cooperative Agreement No. 18-C-99490/3-01 from the Health Care Financing Administration and by the Professional Development Award Program of Research Triangle Institute. The authors acknowledge the support of Toni Pickard, HCFA Project Officer, and the research assistance of Meri Beth Stegall and Meg Johantgen. The opinions expressed are those of the authors and should not be construed as those of the project sponsors.

Chapter 1

Lessons from a Decade of Diffusion and Confusion

Legislation

Medicaid was established in 1965 through Title XIX of the Social Security Act as the federal-state program to finance health care for low-income persons. Although the program's growth was moderate initially, Medicaid experienced serious and accelerated growth in expenditures during the 1980s (see Figure 1.1). This period also witnessed attempts at controlling these expenditures that were unprecedented in their variety and pervasiveness. Much of this variety was set in motion by the passage of the Omnibus Budget Reconciliation Act (OBRA) of 1981. OBRA was critical in encouraging states, through the program waiver application process, to develop new initiatives to both curb costs and improve the delivery and payment mechanisms in use in Medicaid. Subject to the discretionary approval of the Health Care Financing Administration (HCFA), states were permitted to depart from legislative and regulatory provisions governing Medicaid, as contained in Title XIX of the Social Security Act and its various amendments.

This book explores the accumulated experience from one set of the Medicaid reform initiatives ushered in with the OBRA legislation—those relating to primary care case management (PCCM). Medicaid PCCM represents a set of managed care strategies[1] that offer the Medicaid beneficiary access to a primary care provider, who either provides services directly or authorizes referral or specialty services. One set of PCCM programs reimburses the provider on a fee-for-service (FFS) basis; we refer to this as the FFS gatekeeper model. A second set of PCCM programs uses networks of physicians who are capitated or at other financial risk. The third set of PCCM programs involves the enrollment of Medicaid beneficiaries in

Figure 1.1 Growth of Medicaid Expenditures, 1966–1991

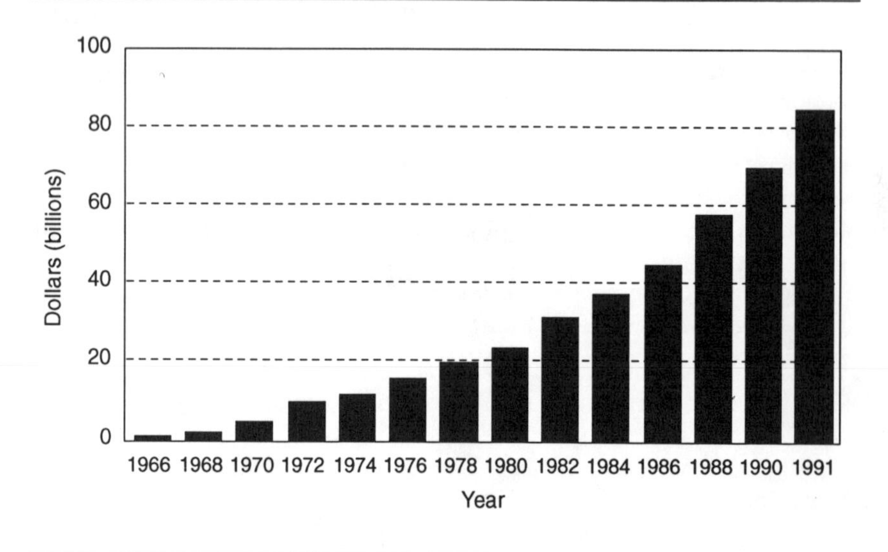

Source: General Accounting Office.

health maintenance organizations (HMOs) or other prepaid health plans (PHPs).[2] A typology of Medicaid PCCM is fully developed in Chapter 4.

Although a limited number of these programs had been initiated under the preexisting research and demonstration waivers (Section 1115 waivers), the rapid expansion of PCCM programs was promoted by the new waiver-granting authority (Section 1915b) that came with OBRA. The PCCM strategy is important for several reasons, including

- its widespread use;
- the many programmatic manifestations;
- important cost, access, and quality implications;
- the potential impact on provider participation in Medicaid;
- controversial restrictions on beneficiary choice of provider;
- its similarity to initiatives under way in the private sector; and
- the substantial investment of funds by federal and state governments in evaluating these programs.

After a decade of PCCM experience and evidence, it is now both possible and desirable to provide a comprehensive appraisal of this strategy, which has witnessed both significant diffusion and confusion. Furthermore, this examination is timely, given the state of flux of health care in the United States, the ongoing debate over its future, and the interest in managed care options, such as PCCM, that the debate has generated.

The initial wave of Medicaid PCCM programs began in 1981 and 1982. Section 1115 waiver authority encouraged variation and creativity. The early programs embodied innovative features that included PCCM as well as capitation payments, restrictions on freedom of choice, competition, and local modifications to state Medicaid programs. As the early descriptive literature reported, accommodating influential participants resulted in an even greater program variety than many developers intended or desired (Hurley 1986). Given the lack of precedent and a relative freedom in program design, the first generation of programs was highly idiosyncratic.

Number and Diversity of Programs

The number of Medicaid managed care programs and the number of states developing them grew throughout most of the decade, as shown in Figure 1.2. As described in detail in later chapters, the engine for the growth in the later part of the decade has largely been PCCM programs.

For several years the development of managed care in Medicaid was chronicled by the National Governors' Association (NGA), which pro-

Figure 1.2 Growth of Medicaid Managed Care, 1981–1992

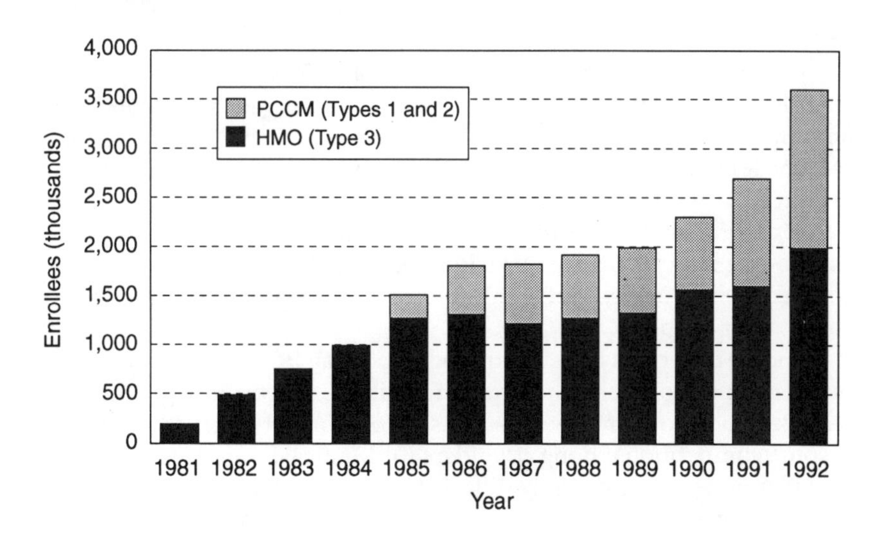

Source: HCFA.

duced an embryonic classification system and played an important catalytic and cross-fertilizing role for the early generation of programs. By 1986 a study using NGA data identified a total of 129 individual participating plans in 25 states (Freund and Neuschler 1986). Hurley and Freund (1988) reported that more than half of the states by that time had developed some form of PCCM. Over 3.6 million beneficiaries were in some form of PCCM by June 1991, and the number of individual plans had increased to 235.

A notable consequence of this expansion was that late entrants have been able to examine a variety of operational models prior to adopting their own preferred approach. Even though developers have not always exploited the available experience, some have gone so far as to conduct on-site visits and systematic appraisals of the importability of a particular model into a prospective site or locale. An example of this is the Michigan Physician Sponsors Plan, which was established in 1982 and was described in Freund's 1984 book of four case studies of primary care management in Medicaid. The state of Kansas patterned its FFS gatekeeper model directly after the Michigan program. In 1985 program developers in Kentucky modeled the Kentucky Patient Access and Care system (KenPAC) after the Kansas program, making KenPAC one generation removed from the original Michigan model. The developers of the North Carolina FFS gatekeeper program, in turn, relied heavily on the KenPAC model during their program design. Further diffusion of the model continues in such states as Virginia, Maryland, and Massachusetts. In 1991 both Massachusetts and New York passed legislation mandating the enrollment of Medicaid beneficiaries in managed care plans. Medicaid PCCM is an important part of the initiatives in these states.

Despite the growth and diffusion of PCCM experience, understanding of the implications of this strategy has lagged, and a substantial amount of confusion about PCCM has been evident. There are many reasons for this confusion. One is that the encouragement of variation has produced a wide assortment of programmatic models, making comparisons difficult. Models have differed in important characteristics, such as sponsorship, structure, provider participation, provider payment, covered beneficiaries, and a number of other features as described in subsequent chapters.

Some observers have attempted to portray PCCM as one of a series of procompetition cost-containment initiatives, even though the competitive dimensions of these programs are obscure, at best. Although there is some competition among providers for Medicaid enrollees in terms of provider networks and mildly differing benefit packages, there have been few if any of the typical demand-side incentives usually discussed in competitive contexts. Only minimal copayments for services are permitted.

Other portrayals of PCCM have failed to disentangle the concept of case management from the use of capitation or other forms of risk sharing. When these features are used in tandem, as has frequently been the case, it is analytically difficult to attribute effects to one or the other feature. Likewise, the distinctions between individual physician case management and prepaid organization-based case management, such as that found in HMOs, often have not been made clear, compounding the difficult job for the analyst.

In the first-generation programs, the duties of PCCM physicians often were unspecified, suggesting that whatever was observed could not be linked explicitly to PCCM. Early critics saw this omission, in conjunction with restrictions on beneficiary freedom of choice, as an invitation to impeded access and to underservice. Other opponents saw the use of structures such as health insuring organizations (HIOs) that used PCCM as unacceptable attempts by states to privatize Medicaid and vacate public responsibility. More generally, the lack of program uniformity permitted (and even promoted) by the waiver process caused concern about equity and equality of access. The early waiver applications often were lacking in rigorously analyzed data that could allay such concerns, a problem that still persists.

Research and Evaluation

A number of substantial and well-performed evaluations that had to confront the problems of variation and asymmetry in program designs were undertaken during this period. The three most extensive of these—the Medicaid Competition Demonstration (MCD) evaluation (RTI 1989), the Medicaid Program Evaluation (MPE) (ORD 1987), and the Arizona Health Care Cost Containment System (AHCCCS) Evaluation (SRI International 1989)—provide an important foundation of descriptive and analytical information from more than a dozen different programs. However, no attempt was made to either integrate or synthesize the findings from these evaluations. Several other states commissioned independent assessments, but few of them made an effort to link their findings to those of other programs. Likewise, it was only in the final years of the decade that descriptive, conceptual, and empirical work from the many programs reached the health services and health policy literature and thus a wide audience of policymakers, program developers, and researchers.

Plan for the Book

This book explicitly addresses the absence of integrated and synthesized evidence from the past decade of experience with PCCM in Medicaid. A general model for PCCM with hypothesized effects on cost and utilization is presented in Chapter 2. The rationales for and approaches to implementing the primary care management strategy for Medicaid-eligible populations are delineated in Chapter 3. A typology developed by Hurley and Freund (1988) is used in Chapter 4 to classify programs on key features and to identify commonalities and differences across programs. Three broad program prototypes that demonstrate the principal models present in PCCM for Medicaid beneficiaries are derived. The design features of 25 programs in 16 states are examined and classified in Chapter 5, using the typology and the derived prototypes.

From the classification of programs, evidence is evaluated in Chapter 6 regarding effects on cost and use in the 25 programs. Assessing the evidence is critical, given the differing sources and varying validity of the findings from the programs. Informed by the findings for each program, impact evidence is summarized by both individual program design features and by the three program prototypes. Chapter 7 presents conclusions from the evidence and implications for both policy and program design. Finally, Chapter 8 concludes with a discussion of areas that require further research. In addition to references, a select bibliography of published post-OBRA PCCM literature is included, along with an appendix containing a synopsis of each of the 25 programs comprising the study population for this study.

Notes

1. Managed care includes, but is not limited to, strategies for controlling costs and improving access that focus on primary care and prepaid arrangements as an alternative to traditional, FFS-based, retrospective reimbursement of costs.
2. We use the term "PHP" to represent more generic models of organizations receiving prepayment for a full range of services. Some PHPs are licensed entities that qualify as HMOs.

References

Freund, D. 1984. *Medicaid Reform: Four Studies of Case Management.* Washington, DC: American Enterprise Institute.

Freund, D., and E. Neuschler. 1986. "Overview of Medicaid Capitation and Case Management Initiatives." *Health Care Financing Review* (Annual Supplement): 21–30.

Health Care Financing Administration (HCFA). 1992. "Medicaid Coordinated Care Enrollment Report: Summary Statistics as of June 30, 1992." Medicaid Bureau.

Hurley, R. 1986. "Status of the Medicaid Competition Demonstrations." *Health Care Financing Review* 8(2): 65–75.

Hurley, R., and D. Freund. 1988. "A Typology of Medicaid Managed Care." *Medical Care* 26(8): 764–73.

Office of Research and Demonstration (ORD). 1987. *Medicaid Program Evaluation: Final Report.* Report No. MPE 9.2. Eds. J. Holahan, J. Bell, and G. S. Adler. Baltimore, MD: Health Care Financing Administration.

Research Triangle Institute (RTI). 1989. *Evaluation of the Medicaid Competition Demonstrations: Integrative Final Report.* Contract No. HCFA-500-83-0050. Research Triangle Park, NC: Research Triangle Institute.

SRI International. 1989. *Evaluation of the Arizona Health Care Cost Containment System: Final Report.* Contract No. HCFA-500-83-0027. Palo Alto, CA: SRI International.

Chapter 2

The Transformation from Primary Care Management to Primary Care Gatekeeping

The diversity of PCCM programs can be neither understood nor evaluated without an appreciation of the evolution of primary care in the United States. The primary care physician (PCP) plays a pivotal role in the U.S. health care system. This role has long been recognized and was significantly reinvigorated by the development of family medicine as a specialty in the late 1960s. At the heart of the advocacy for primary care medicine is the importance of ready access to broadly prepared, versatile clinicians in an increasingly specialized, technologically sophisticated delivery environment. Implicitly, the argument has been a clinical one: Caring and curing can be better if PCPs are in the front lines of service provision and management.

By the late 1970s a new interpretation of primary care management, now commonly called primary care case management (PCCM) or primary care gatekeeping, emerged. The PCP was additionally being credited with the capacity to make a significant cost-containment contribution. Many of the clinical virtues of care by a PCP were asserted to have economic value as well. The availability of a PCP could divert care from more expensive sources; continuity in care could improve efficiency as well as quality; redundancy in ancillary use could be reduced if care were concentrated with fewer providers. Moreover, it was argued that PCPs have, in effect, been gatekeeping access to specialists and inpatient care all along. Both of these services are substantially more expensive than primary care and possibly even avoidable if primary care providers and their patients can be induced to use less costly alternatives.

Also in this decade there was a dramatic proliferation of public and private sector PCCM programs. While Medicaid has been a major promoter of this approach, 93 percent of HMOs report using primary care gatekeeping as a cost-control strategy (GHAA 1989). More recently, the use of gatekeeping has become common in preferred provider organizations (PPOs) and so-called point-of-service delivery systems that are hybrids of HMOs and PPOs (Boland 1991). These gatekeeping programs share a common strategy to transform the primary care clinician into a cost-conscious allocator of health service resources.

The discussion of the transformation of primary care management into PCCM begins with a definition and specification of goals. The parallel transition of clinical dimensions and economic characteristics is described. Further, a model of contemporary primary care gatekeeping is presented from which a series of hypothesized program effects is delineated.

Definition and Goals

Under PCCM, a beneficiary (patient) is enrolled with a PCP or an organization with primary care capacity. The physician or organization assumes explicit responsibility to provide, arrange, or authorize all covered non-emergency medical care. Care not provided by or authorized for the enrollee by the gatekeeper will not be compensated by the beneficiary's insurer or sponsor. The physician-gatekeeper promises continuous, 24-hour availability in person or through arrangements to (1) perform these duties and (2) ensure the enrollee will have access when needed. When the enrollment is with an organization rather than with an individual physician, the enrollee should be able to identify a specific physician who is the principal point of contact for service and authorization.

The goals of primary care gatekeeping programs are customarily expressed as twofold: cost-effectiveness and ensured access.

The first of these goals, cost-effectiveness, is anchored in the belief that this form of service delivery can minimize the resources consumed in rendering required medical services. This goal implies that the PCCM strategy is clinically and economically superior to fragmented and discontinuous care not coordinated by a responsible, informed primary care practitioner. Moreover, promoting (mandating) a sustained relationship with a PCP can strengthen the relational dimensions of the care delivery process that are believed to improve outcomes, including greater patient satisfaction. The formal linkage of physician and patient can also heighten a physician's sense of accountability to his or her enrollees and thereby encourage high-quality performance. Finally, the goal of ensuring access is attained by the formal commitment the physician-gatekeeper makes to be continuously available to enrollees.

The essential aim of primary care gatekeeping programs is to provide the benefits of primary care management to an enrolled population. These programs do so by securing an explicit, contractual agreement from a physician to perform specified primary care management functions. It is important to note that the definition and goals of primary care gatekeeping make no statements about how gatekeepers are paid. Payment methods may be viewed as optional incentives and disincentives that can be used to intensify pressure on gatekeepers to attain some of these goals.

The appeal of the primary care gatekeeping strategy is likely to be strongest when past achievement of its goals has been problematic. If access has been constrained, gatekeeping can be an effective approach to overcoming impediments. If quality of care has been questionable, enhanced accountability and monitoring of performance under PCCM will be highly desirable. In systems of care where the lack of a sustained relationship has been a source of discontinuity and dissatisfaction (e.g., in emergency departments or in early prepaid group practice settings), formal linkage with an identified personal physician can address this problem. Finally, where inefficient patterns of use or an excessive level of utilization have been experienced, gatekeeping can be an especially attractive cost-control remedy.

The Case for Primary Care Management

The principal functions of primary care providers have been described as (1) providing first contact care, (2) assuming longitudinal responsibility for health and illness, and (3) coordinating the use of the health care system, especially visits to specialists (Alpert and Charney 1973). The Institute of Medicine (1977) identified five attributes as essential to the practice of good primary care medicine: accessibility, comprehensiveness, coordination, continuity, and accountability.

These attributes originally were specified as critical to providing high-quality care but subsequently have been recognized to have significant economic implications as well.

After several decades of precipitous decline in the numbers of PCPs (White 1964; Citizens' Commission 1966; National Commission 1966; Stevens and Stevens 1974; Starr 1982; Moore and Priebe 1991), renewed interest in the mid-1970s led to the development of the family medicine specialty. Health care services were viewed as increasingly fragmented, impersonal, disease-oriented, and costly (Lewis 1976). The decline in the importance of the relational aspects of medical care relative to the technological sophistication of the physician was seen as having significant negative implications.

The case for primary care medicine and primary care management was built both on ideology and on empirical evidence from studies on continuity and comprehensiveness in care (Ad Hoc Committee on the Education for Family Practice of the Council on Medical Education 1966). For example, continuous patient-provider relationships had been found to be associated with enhanced patient disclosure of information (Hill 1964; Becker, Drachman, and Kirscht 1974b) and improved patient compliance with medical regimens (Becker, Stolley, and Lasagna 1972; Poland 1976; Stokes 1980; Charney et al. 1967; Fink et al. 1969). Other specific clinical benefits of continuity of medical care that were found included reduced discomfort and reduced levels of disability (Gordis and Markowitz 1971; Alpert et al. 1968).

Perhaps the most consistently demonstrated finding regarding the impact of continuity was a positive correlation with patient satisfaction. This result was apparent across a variety of studies that employed many different measures of continuity (Alpert et al. 1968; Becker, Drachman, and Kirscht 1974a and 1974b; Caplan and Sussman 1966; Shortell 1976; Shortell et al. 1977; Woolley et al. 1978). Continuous care also has been found to have a positive influence on patient attitudes about the quality of the care received, the knowledge and attitudes of their providers, and health beliefs (Becker, Drachman, and Kirscht 1974c). Provider satisfaction was found to be higher in continuous patient-provider relationships (Becker, Drachman, and Kirscht 1974b; Sussman and Haug 1969; Haegarty et al. 1970; Becker, Stolley, and Lasagna 1972; Caplan and Sussman 1966; Rockart and Hofmann 1969).

Primary care management was also asserted to contribute to more efficient use of medical resources. Continuity in the provider relationship enables the physician to more expeditiously and proficiently recognize medical problems and prescribe treatments appropriate to his or her particular patients. This continuity has been shown to result in fewer laboratory tests and procedures (Starfield et al. 1976; Hennelly and Boxerman 1979), fewer illness visits (Alpert et al. 1968; Breslau and Haug 1976; Gordis and Markowitz 1971; Haegerty et al. 1970; Hennelly and Boxerman 1979; Roos, et al. 1980), and fewer emergency hospitalizations (Haegarty et al. 1970).

In addition to the benefits of improved coordination of care, the use of primary care providers as a patient's initial point of entry into the medical care system affords other opportunities for economizing on care. When compared to specialists, PCPs have been found to order fewer laboratory tests (Scherger et al. 1980; Noren et al. 1980; Smith and McWhinney 1975). Prescribing habits and medication selection by PCPs also differ from that of specialists (Schroeder 1980). Primary care physicians also have a lower likelihood of making referrals for specialty consultations, reflecting their greater versatility and self-reliance (Perkoff 1978). Freidson eloquently described the "elasticity of referral boundaries" (1975) when he discussed how PCPs in a prepaid group practice exercised discretion over the conditions and procedures they determined to be within or beyond their domain of competence.

The rediscovery of the virtues of primary care medicine occurred at the same time that concern about cost containment among all purchasers of health care began growing. Economists such as Fuchs (1974) and Enthoven (1978) both emphasized the key purchasing agent role of the physician-gatekeeper. Given the sparse but notable evidence supporting the economic benefits of primary care management, cost concerns became connected with the fundamental clinical (and political) appeal of expanded availability of primary care. The most attractive aspect of this connection was the argument that cost containment could be achieved by expanding access to primary care. Consequently, the primary care management strategy also appeared to be a model of allocative efficiency.

Moore's noteworthy article on the SAFECO United Healthcare program in 1979 is the benchmark for the modern era of primary care gatekeeping. He not only explicitly linked primary care management and gatekeeping but also provided a succinct summary of the underlying logic of this strategy:

> . . . to the extent that primary care physicians are likely to use less expensive medical technology, fewer procedures and less surgical treatment for initial management of common problems, costs are lower than if patients went to specialists for initial management. Moreover, the continuity of care provided by one coordinating physician is likely to reduce unnecessary duplication of diagnostic tests and therapeutic trials, thereby increasing the efficiency of the entire health care system. (Moore 1979, p. 1362)

While not responsive to all aspects of cost containment, primary care management offers a reasonable and, importantly, professionally acceptable approach to tackling the intractable health care cost issue.

Gatekeeper Effects on Patient Care
A Conceptual Model

The search for cost-containment strategies in the 1970s and 1980s led to the office door of the PCP. Recognizing the physician as the principal purchasing agent for the health care delivery system, insurers and other payers concluded that if this pivotal care management position could be promoted, and perhaps exploited, cost-containment goals could be made consonant with optimal care goals. The PCP could be permitted to be an effective care manager and induced, either directly or indirectly, to also be an efficient cost manager. The question became, How could the apparent clinical advantages of primary care management be turned into an economic advantage as well? The answer was to enlist the PCP to assume formally the role of primary care gatekeeper.

Two features of the PCP as gatekeeper distinguish this role from the traditional primary care manager role. The first distinction lies in the gatekeeper's assumption of what can be called utilization management responsibilities, including the acceptance of payer-imposed performance standards and feedback. Gatekeeping PCPs agree to exercise discretion in decisions affecting resources consumed by their patients and to have their performance monitored in this regard. The gatekeeper responsibility also includes formally agreeing to be continuously available to provide primary care services and to authorize judiciously all referral care. Aggressive substitution of less costly alternative treatment regimens can be another condition of participation. The acceptance and observance of specified diagnostic and treatment protocols is a third type of imposed responsibility. In each case, gatekeepers are monitored for adherence to performance standards within specified tolerance levels.

The second distinguishing feature of gatekeeping is the restriction on provider choice for patients/enrollees, which in effect imposes regimentation on their health care–seeking patterns. This dimension channels patients to their gatekeepers, thereby enabling the gatekeeper to provide care directly and to perform utilization management functions.

The mandatory (locked-in) nature of this relationship has several implications. Gatekeepers are likely to feel a heightened sense of professional responsibility to their patients (as well as increased potential for conflicts of interest). Patient patterns of use inevitably are altered by the suppression of self-referring behavior. As needed, the patient is routed to members of the gatekeeper's referral network. Primary care physician relationships with referral sources of care might be changed by virtue of the empowerment of the PCP via the gatekeeper authority. In a somewhat more subtle but important sense, the external accountability of physicians for their performance is enhanced by the enrollment of patients whose cost and use experience and, arguably, well-being, can now be attributed to their gatekeeping. At the very least, the enrolled patients become the denominator used in the calculation of gatekeeper-specific performance statistics.

A general model of the cumulative effect of primary care management and primary care management with gatekeeping is illustrated in Figures 2.1, 2.2, and 2.3. In Figure 2.1, the patient has free access to primary care service providers and may self-refer for specialist care, to the extent such providers will see patients on self-referral. Within the total care boundary, care is neither formally managed nor coordinated by anyone other than the care-seeker. In Figure 2.2, into which primary care management has been introduced, the patient chooses to affiliate with a PCP who, by mutual

Figure 2.1 Medical Care with No Primary Care Management

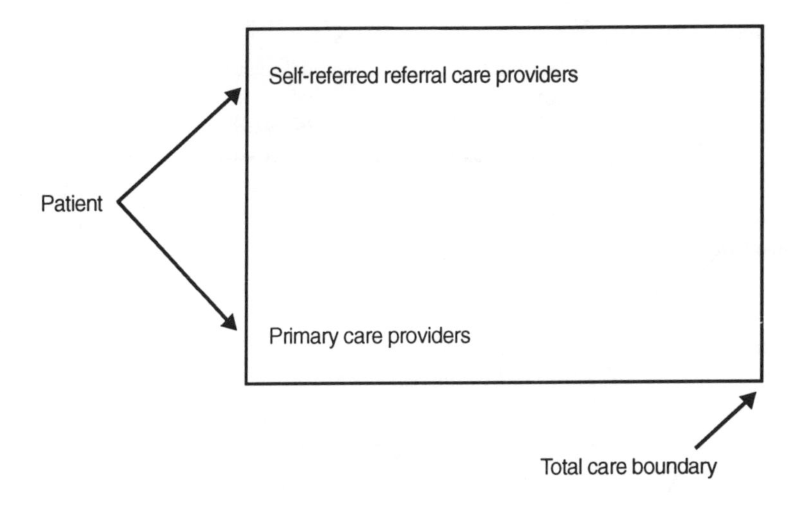

Figure 2.2 Medical Care with Primary Care Management

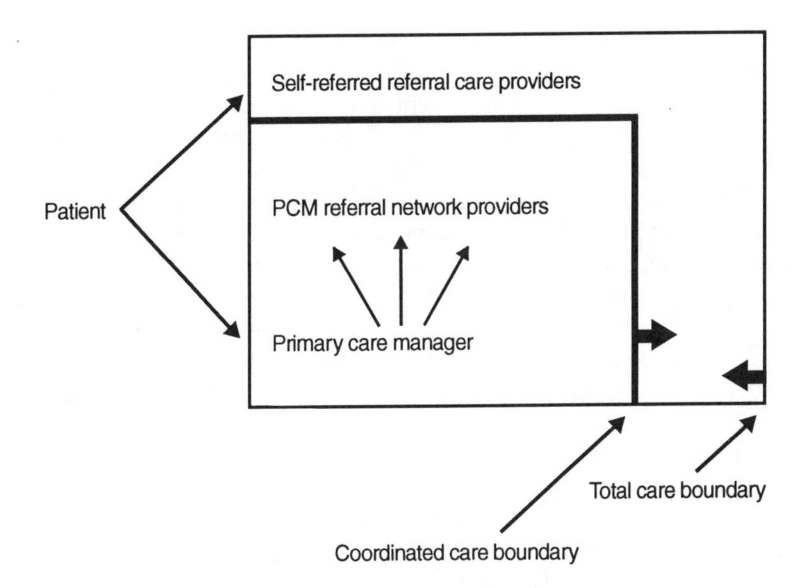

agreement with the patient, directly renders necessary care. As a primary care manager, the PCP also provides access to a preexisting referral network that becomes the source of a substantial portion of the previously self-referred or, at the least, uncoordinated care. Consequently, the patient

Figure 2.3 Medical Care with Primary Care Management and Gatekeeping

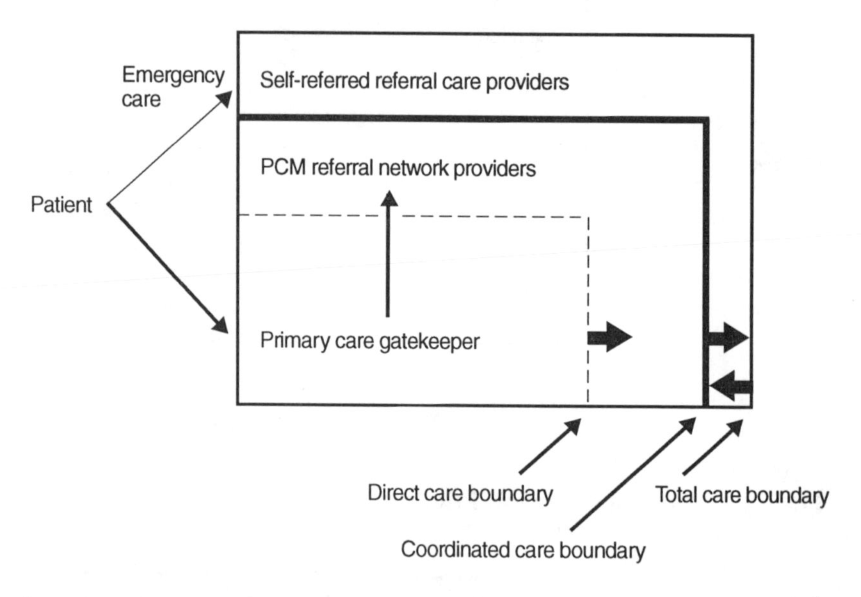

decreases the extent of self-referring behavior in proportion to confidence in and dependence on the judgment of the PCP.

The coordinated care boundary refers to the portion of total care that is subject to management by the PCP. The establishment of a sustained patient–primary care manager relationship brings to bear the benefits of familiarity and longitudinality. Integral parts of this relationship include the primary care manager's implicit agreement to be available on an as-needed basis to affiliated patients and to accept professional responsibility for care management and coordination. This responsibility typically is manifested in both increased concentration of directly provided care and improved process continuity (concentration and coordination) during episodes of illness. Finally, the primary care manager becomes the repository for a unit medical record in which all pertinent data are consolidated.

The implications of adding the two gatekeeping dimensions to the primary care manager role are shown in Figure 2.3. The choice-restricting, lock-in feature (solid line) restricts all but true emergency care to the primary care manager. This feature virtually eliminates self-referred care, as it forces all specialist care to come through the primary care manager's own referral network. In effect the coordinated care boundary moves toward being coterminous with the total care boundary. However, the impact of the utilization management responsibility is potentially more complex. It can reduce the entire amount of care obtained by the patient under gatekeeping by shrinking the total care boundary. The total amount of care received through the referral network can be reduced by the denial of referrals or by the substitution of care by the primary care manager for specialist or referral care. Implicitly this represents a shift in the domain of the primary care manager's range of practice or scope of services (i.e., an outward expansion of the direct care boundary), demonstrating the elasticity of referral behavior suggested by Freidson (1975).

This model of gatekeeping suggests that its goal is to force the direct care boundary toward the coordinated care boundary, and in turn the coordinated care boundary toward the total care boundary, so that virtually all care becomes managed. The limiting case is that all necessary care, and no additional care, be provided by the primary care manager–gatekeeper, as long as the primary care manager judges the care to lie within his or her realm of competence. Standards and targets may be developed by gatekeeping sponsors to encourage primary care manager–gatekeepers to conform their practice patterns to specified performance expectations.

As described in Chapter 4, a variety of payment methods have been used to compensate the primary care gatekeeper. These methods range from FFS to capitation for primary care services with the opportunity to share in savings from reduced referral services. The model of gatekeeping proposed above suggests that the role of financial incentives and inducements should be viewed as intensifying pressure on gatekeepers to perform rigorously their utilization management functions. For example, financially at-risk gatekeepers might more vigorously pursue the substitution of less costly services for more costly, clinically equivalent services. This example is not to say that FFS gatekeeping will not have detectable effects on, for instance, beneficiary cost and use; the model suggests it might. However, these effects may be more substantial when financial incentives are employed.

Applying the Conceptual Model: Selected Hypotheses

The model attempts to present a comprehensive picture of the effects of primary care gatekeeping. However, given the limited data available from the selected programs examined in this study, and the focus solely on use and cost effects, it is necessary to narrow the scope of the hypotheses proposed for testing to the following areas: physician visits, emergency department visits, ancillary and prescription use, inpatient use, and total expenditures for covered services. Other important areas, such as satisfaction and quality of care, cannot be explicitly addressed in this study as too few evaluations have performed serious assessments of quality.[1]

The discussion of hypothesized effects under PCCM begins with the type of utilization most likely to be influenced—physician visits—and proceeds through to the aggregate effects of gatekeeping as manifested in total resources consumed or service expenditures.

Physician visits

The conceptual model suggests that the dynamics of primary care gatekeeping might affect the use of physician services in several ways. First of all, if the enrollee had problems in obtaining access to care in the past, the guaranteed availability of a source of primary care could lead to increased use of physician services. There is also the possibility of decreases in use for the patient who has had access to care but not to a usual source of care. Additionally, there is a likelihood of a reduction in the number of specialist visits by enrollees, in part because of the suppression of self-referrals and in part (perhaps) because of more judicious decision making by gatekeepers regarding specialist use. It is possible, however, that reductions in specialist referrals are offset by expanded numbers of visits to the PCP. This response would be consistent with a shifting of the direct care boundary toward the coordinated care boundary. Finally, the method by which primary care gatekeepers are compensated, including opportunities to share in savings resulting from reduced specialist use, might influence overall volume of physician visits.

Based on the conflicting and countervailing pressures on gatekeepers, we hypothesize the following impact for physician visits.

Hypothesis 1: The effect of primary care gatekeeping on utilization will be mixed and will depend on the payment mechanism.

Hypothesis 1a: Under FFS the effect of primary care gatekeeping will be to increase the total number of physician visits.

Hypothesis 1b: If physicians are paid on an at-risk basis the effect of primary care gatekeeping will be to decrease the total number of physician visits.

For a limited number of programs, the dynamics of gatekeeping have been studied at the visit level by physician specialty (Long and Settle 1988; Hurley, Freund, and Gage 1991), but visit-level detail is not available from most of the programs we examined in this study.

Emergency department visits

Primary care gatekeeping is expected to sharply reduce the use of hospital and freestanding emergency departments, especially for Medicaid beneficiaries who have grown to rely on this site as a source of continuously available primary care. As shown in Figure 2.3, all nonemergency care is channeled to the primary care gatekeeper for provision or authorization. Gatekeeper programs typically require emergency department staff to contact primary care gatekeepers if one of their enrollees presents for a visit that is not a true emergency.

It is more likely, however, that the enrollment with a PCP who guarantees to be continuously available is the factor that reduces demand for emergency department services among beneficiaries. Some of these reductions in emergency department use might be offset by office visits to the gatekeeper, or by simple telephone contacts for reassurance or guidance from a PCP knowledgeable about the beneficiaries and their medical history and needs.

Hypothesis 2: Emergency department use will be lower under all gatekeeper program designs because of a guaranteed relationship with a PCP and because emergency department visits for other than true emergencies will not be reimbursed unless formally authorized by the gatekeeper.

Ancillary care and prescription use

Anchoring an enrollee-patient with a primary care gatekeeper who coordinates virtually all care and who must authorize any referral care offers an opportunity to reduce redundancy and repetition in the provision of diagnostic and therapeutic services. Primary care physicians develop relationships with their patients and develop cumulative and unified medical records for them. Since referral care must be explicitly authorized by gatekeepers, specialists can be readily informed regarding past work-ups and findings, without necessarily having to repeat them. Results of specialty consultations are also returned to the patients' "medical home" and incorporated into the centralized medical record. Improved gatekeeper-directed coordination of care can also reduce the use of multiple and potentially negatively synergistic prescriptions among beneficiaries. Because care coordination represents an important aspect of utilization management, it is likely that offering financial incentives to gatekeepers might induce them to manage more rigorously any resources expended in this area.

Hypothesis 3: Ancillary and prescription use will be lower in gatekeeper programs.

Hypothesis 3a: In PCCM programs that place gatekeepers at financial risk, ancillary and prescription use will be even lower.

Inpatient use

The proposed model of primary care gatekeeping does not directly address whether inpatient use will be altered for beneficiaries enrolled with gatekeepers. If it is assumed that some admissions or days of care are due to a lack of coordination of care or to the inadequate use of alternatives to inpatient services, then some reduction in inpatient use might be observed among enrollees. More generally, if a primary care relationship fosters more use of preventive services and promotes healthy behaviors, then gatekeeping could have the impact of ultimately avoiding some inpatient use. In either case, it is likely that the impact of gatekeeping on inpatient use would be relatively modest but could be intensified if the gatekeeper were at some financial risk.

A potentially confounding factor in examining the effect of primary care gatekeeping and inpatient use is that sponsors of gatekeeping might accompany the initiatives with other utilization management mechanisms that specifically target inpatient use, such as preadmission certification and concurrent inpatient review. These mechanisms can be integral parts of cost-containment interventions but should conceptually be kept separate from the gatekeeper component.

An additional factor relating to inpatient effects relates to the basic health needs of the populations subject to PCCM. In the case of Medicaid, many of the programs focus solely on Aid to Families with Dependent Children (AFDC) beneficiaries. Childbirth is the primary reason for hospital admissions for this group. It is unlikely that PCCM would significantly affect numbers of admissions for this group; it could, however, affect length of stay (LOS) through better prenatal care and subsequent prevention of low-birthweight babies.

Hypothesis 4: Inpatient use will be unchanged or slightly lower in primary gatekeeper programs due to better care coordination.

Hypothesis 4a: PCCM programs with financially at-risk gatekeepers and PHPs are more likely to reduce inpatient use.

Beneficiary health care costs

The hypothesized impacts described above relating to physician, emergency department, ancillary, and inpatient use suggest that total health care expenditures will be affected by primary care gatekeeping. The reductions in volume of care can produce expenditure reductions even without price reductions for individual services, which is not a reasonable option for most Medicaid programs. It is worth noting, however, that gatekeeping programs do allow the opportunity to extract price concessions because of the potential for channeling and guaranteeing patient volumes to gatekeepers and referral network providers. Because we hypothesized that selected service utilization will be reduced more through the use of financial incentives, total expenditures will be correspondingly affected.

Hypothesis 5: Primary care gatekeeper programs will result in small but significant reductions in overall program expenditures.

Hypothesis 5a: Expenditures may be larger in PCCM programs that employ financial risk-sharing with the gatekeepers.

To reiterate, the hypotheses we can ultimately test are limited by the availability of data from the 25 Medicaid managed-care programs included in this study. However, several other implications of primary care gatekeeping, beyond the scope of the data available for this study, are discussed in Chapter 8. Among these are the impact of PCCM on quality of care, patient and physician satisfaction, relations between primary care and specialist physicians, and provider participation.

Note

1. Note, however, that several of the studies we included have addressed these areas. In particular, the MCD evaluation (RTI 1989) and the AHCCCS evaluation (SRI International 1989) specifically address patient satisfaction and quality of care under PCCM.

References

Ad Hoc Committee on the Education for Family Practice of the Council on Medical Education. 1966. *Meeting the Challenge of Family Practice.* Chicago: American Medical Association.

Alpert, J., and E. Charney. 1973. *The Education of Physicians for Primary Care.* DHEW Publication No. (HRA) 74-3113. Rockville, MD: Bureau of Health Services Research.

Alpert, J., M. Haegarty, L. Robertson, J. Kosa, and R. Haggerty. 1968. "Effective Use of Comprehensive Pediatric Care." *American Journal of Diseases of Children* 116: 529–33.

Becker, M. H., R. Drachman, and J. P. Kirscht. 1974a. "Continuity Pediatrician: New Support for an Old Shibboleth." *Journal of Pediatrics* 84(4): 599–605.

———. 1974b. "A Field Experiment to Evaluate Various Outcomes of Continuity of Care." *American Journal of Public Health* 64(11): 1062–70.

———. 1974c. "Predicting Mother's Compliance with Pediatric Medical Regimens." *Journal of Pediatrics* 81: 843–54.

Becker, M., P. Stolley, and L. Lasagna. 1972. "Differential Education Concerning Therapeutics and Resulting Prescribing Patterns." *Journal of Medical Education* 47(2): 118–27.

Boland, P. 1991. *Making Managed Care Work: A Practical Guide to Strategies and Solutions.* New York: McGraw-Hill.

Breslau, N., and M. Haug. 1976. "Service Delivery Structure and Continuity of Care: A Case Study of a Pediatric Practice in Process of Reorganization." *Journal of Health and Social Behavior* 17: 339–52.

Caplan, E., and M. Sussman. 1966. "Rank Order of Important Variables for Patient and Staff Satisfaction with Outpatient Service." *Journal of Health and Human Behavior* 2(7): 133–37.

Charney, E., R. Bynum, D. Eldredge, D. Frank, J. B. MacWhinney, N. McNabb, A. Scheiner, E. A. Sumpler, and H. Iker. 1967. "How Well Do Patients Take Oral Penicillin? A Collaborative Study in Private Practice." *Pediatrics* 40(2): 188–95.

Citizens' Commission on Graduate Medical Education (Millis Commission). 1966. *The Graduate Education of Physicians.* Chicago: American Medical Association.

Enthoven, A. 1978. "Consumer-Choice Health Plan." First of two parts, "Inflation and Inequity in Health Care Today: Alternatives for Cost Control and an Analysis of Proposals for National Health Insurance." *New England Journal of Medicine* 298(12): 650–58.

Fink, D., M. Malloy, M. Cohen, M. Greycloud, and F. Martin. 1969. "Effective Patient Care in the Pediatric Ambulatory Setting: A Study of the Acute Care Clinic." *Pediatrics* 43(6): 927–35.

Freidson, E. 1975. *Doctoring Together: A Study in Profession Social Control.* New York: Elsevier.

Fuchs, V. 1974. *Who Shall Live?* New York: Basic Books.

Gordis, L., and M. Markowitz. 1971. "Evaluation of the Effectiveness of Comprehensive and Continuous Pediatric Care." *Pediatrics* 48(5): 766–76.

Group Health Association of America (GHAA). 1989. *HMO Industry Profile.* Washington, DC: The Association.

Haegarty, M., L. Robertson, J. Kosa, and J. Alpert. 1970. "Some Comparative Costs of Comprehensive Versus Fragmented Pediatric Care." *Pediatrics* 48(4): 596–603.

Hennelly, V., and S. B. Boxerman. 1979. "Continuity of Medical Care: Its Impact on Physician Utilization." *Medical Care* 17: 1012–18.

Hill, M. 1964. "Can Health Be Taught?" *Journal of the Royal Health Society* 84: 125–27.

Hurley, R., D. Freund, and B. Gage. 1991. "Gatekeeper Effects on Patterns of Physician Use." *The Journal of Family Practice* 32(2): 167–74.

Institute of Medicine. 1977. *A Manpower Policy for Primary Health Care.* Washington, DC: National Academy of Sciences.

Lewis, C. 1976. "Does Comprehensive Care Make a Difference? What Is the Evidence?" *American Journal of Diseases of Children* 122: 469–74.

Long, S. and R. Settle. 1988. "An Evaluation of Utah's Primary Care Case Management Program for Medicaid Recipients." *Medical Care* 26(11): 1021–32.

Moore, F. D., and C. Priebe. 1991. "Board Certified Physicians in the United States, 1971–1986." *New England Journal of Medicine* 324(8): 536–43.

Moore, S. 1979. ''Cost Containment Through Risk-Sharing by Primary Care Physicians.'' *New England Journal of Medicine* 300(24): 1359–62.

National Commission on Community Health Services (Folsom Commission). 1966. *Health Is a Community Affair.* Cambridge, MA: Harvard University Press.

Noren, J., T. Frazier, I. Altman, and J. DeLozier. 1980. ''Ambulatory Medical Care: A Comparison of Internists and Family General Practitioners.'' *New England Journal of Medicine* 302(1): 11–16.

Perkoff, G. 1978. ''An Effect of Organization of Medical Care upon Manpower Distribution.''*Medical Care* 16(8): 628–40.

Poland, M. 1976. ''The Effect of Continuity of Care on the Missed Appointment Note in a Prenatal Clinic.'' *Journal of Obstetric, Gynecologic, and Neonatal Nursing* 5: 45.

Research Triangle Institute (RTI). 1989. *Evaluation of the Medicaid Competition Demonstrations: Integrative Final Report.* Contract No. HCFA-500-83-0050. Research Triangle Park, NC: Research Triangle Institute.

Rockart, J. F., and P. Hofmann. 1969. ''Physician and Patient Behavior Under Different Scheduling Systems in a Hospital Outpatient Department.'' *Medical Care* 7(6): 463–70.

Roos, L., N. Roos, P. Gilbert, and J. Nicol. 1980. ''Continuity of Care: Does It Contribute to Quality of Care?'' *Medical Care* 18(2): 174–84.

Scherger, J. E., M. J. Gordon, T. J. Phillips, and J. P. LoGerfro. 1980. ''Comparison of Diagnostic Methods of Family Practice and Internal Medicine Residents.'' *Journal of Family Practice* 10: 96–101.

Schroeder, S. 1980. ''Variations in Physician Practice Patterns: A Review of Medical Cost Implications.'' In *The Physician and Cost Control,* eds. E. Carrels, D. Neuhauser, and W. Stasson, 23–50. Cambridge, MA: Oelgeschlager, Gunn and Hain.

Shortell, S. 1976. ''Continuity of Medical Care: Conceptualization and Measurement.'' *Medical Care* 14(5): 377–91.

Shortell, S., W. Richardson, J. LoGerfo, P. Diehr, B. Weaver, and K. Green. 1977. ''The Relationship Among Dimensions of Health Services in Two Provider Systems: A Causal Model Approach.'' *Journal of Health and Social Behavior* 18: 139–59.

Smith, D., and I. McWhinney. 1975. ''Comparison of the Diagnostic Methods of Family Physicians and Internists.'' *Journal of Medical Education* 50: 264–70.

SRI International. 1989. *Evaluation of the Arizona Health Care Cost Containment System: Final Report.* Contract No. HCFA-500-83-0027. Palo Alto, CA: SRI International.

Starfield, B., D. Simborg, S. Horn, and S. Yourtee. 1976. ''Continuity and Coordination in Primary Care: Their Achievement and Utility.'' *Medical Care* 14(7): 625–36.

Starr, P. 1982. *The Social Transformation of American Medicine.* New York: Basic Books.

Stevens, R. and R. Stevens. 1974. *Welfare Medicine in America.* New York: Free Press.

Stokes, J. 1980. ''Continuous and Comprehensive Patient Care.'' *American Journal of Public Health* 70: 636.

Sussman, M. B., and M. R. Haug. 1969. ''The Vicissitudes of Change.'' *Social Science and Medicine* 3(2): 179–89.

White, K. 1964. "General Practice in the United States." *Journal of Medical Education* 39(4): 344.

Woolley, F., R. Kane, C. Hughes, and D. Wright. 1978. "The Effects of Doctor-Patient Communication on Satisfaction and Outcome of Care." *Social Science and Medicine* 12: 123–28.

Chapter 3

Primary Care Case Management: The Medicaid Context

When the Medicaid program was implemented in 1966 through Title XIX of the Social Security Act, one of its goals was to mimic the private sector system of health insurance (Cohen 1985). The principal implication of this approach was that Medicaid would, like private insurance, essentially be a payment system only and would not attempt to alter or otherwise influence the structure of the existing health care delivery system. The underlying logic was that this approach would minimize resistance to the program and maximize participation among providers of services. In theory, Medicaid patients would receive care and treatment identical with that received by patients covered by other third-party payers.

Among the hallmark features of private insurance in the mid-1960s was the tradition of permitting beneficiaries to have full freedom to choose those providers from whom they wished to receive care. This tradition was problematic in the Medicaid context, however, since Medicaid required participating providers to accept its payment in full (i.e., it did not permit balance billing to beneficiaries as allowed by other insurance programs). This requirement meant Medicaid patients could not choose providers who did not accept payment in full. They could not, in fact, pay the difference out-of-pocket, as Medicare and private insurance beneficiaries could and still do. If Medicaid beneficiaries received care from nonparticipating providers, they were entirely responsible for costs. The main reason for this requirement was that eligible persons were assumed not to have the discretionary income to make such payments, and providers had to be prepared to accept what the Medicaid program would pay. Thus, in practice, this restriction limited access to those individuals and organizations who agreed to be participating providers (i.e., those who would accept the conditions for payment under the Medicaid program).

This divergence from private insurance programs at the time that Medicaid was implemented is noteworthy for two reasons. First, it established an implicit restriction on freedom of choice that would worsen over time as what Medicaid programs *would* pay became entangled in the debate over what Medicaid programs *could* pay. As payment rates have declined over the years in real dollar terms, the level of provider participation has also fallen. This situation has in turn reduced the prerogatives of choice-seeking beneficiaries and ultimately contributed to inefficient and undesirable patterns of health care use. Second, it is noteworthy that the Medicaid approach portended contemporary growth of choice-restricting delivery systems such as preferred provider networks (e.g., PPOs and related entities). The Medicaid approach consisted of contracting with a subset of the universe of potential providers who agreed to accept a discounted third-party payment in full and who also agreed to accept restrictions on their professional autonomy such as prior authorization. It is not an overstatement to suggest that Medicaid was the first preferred (or more aptly, exclusive) provider organization (Hurley and Freund 1988).

Problems in the Medicaid Delivery System

The issue of provider participation in Medicaid has been extensively and thoroughly described (Sloan, Mitchell and Cromwell 1978; Cromwell and Mitchell 1984; Davidson, Cromwell, and Schurman 1986; Perloff, Kletke, and Neckerman 1987). Not only has participation declined in terms of real numbers of providers, careful research has documented that the decline is even more severe when analysis is based on the composition of the practices of those providers who continue to see some Medicaid patients. As Mitchell and Cromwell (1980) have reported, the concentration of Medicaid patients in relatively few provider sites is striking. Moreover, the quality of these providers has frequently been called into question in both clinical and sometimes ethical or legal terms. The term *Medicaid mill* connotes both large throngs of patients, and clinical and billing practices of dubious appropriateness. Despite the frequent claims of fraud and abuse leveled at such providers, it should be emphasized that there is no evidence to suggest that illegal practices are any more widespread in the public than in the private health care sector (Reinhardt 1985). However, problems are certainly more publicized in the former than in the latter.

A particularly pernicious consequence of the shifting of Medicaid-covered care to large institutional providers has been sharp declines in participation by individual physicians. The reasons for this shift are often cited as both economic and sociologic (Perloff, Kletke, and Neckerman 1987), having to do with asserted insufficiency of payments (the two-market theory) and the intolerability of intrusive provisions on physician discretion (the professional autonomy theory). Thus, those providers who continue to participate are commonly viewed as those who cannot replace Medicaid patients in their practices with more desirable private patients or who are prepared to live with restrictions on their autonomy. Continued willingness to participate in Medicaid might be due to financial reasons, geographic location, traditional mission (such as for public hospitals or health centers), or dubious reputation. Although these reasons certainly do not apply in all cases, there has been enough evidence to say that in practice the Medicaid program is far from meeting the theoretical ideal of full freedom of choice of provider.

Medicaid beneficiaries themselves have also been identified as a source of some of the unwillingness of providers to participate in the program. In addition to being financially disadvantaged, eligible populations are commonly undereducated and might manifest values and norms at odds with those of the provider. Moreover, their lifestyles and living conditions are often not conducive to care-seeking patterns comparable to those of majority cultures. All of these factors seem to have contributed to a stereotyped portrait of patients who might be unreliable in keeping appointments, noncompliant, episodic in care seeking, inattentive to changing unhealthy habits, and particularly susceptible to health hazards that most medical providers are ill-equipped to handle effectively. Coupled with the low payments received for their care, this scenario hardly suggests advantages for developing a large Medicaid practice.

The Medicaid Syndrome

The picture of health and medical care that has emerged in 26 years of Medicaid is not a positive one. Chief among the problems and complaints are the following (Freund 1984):

- Restricted access to mainstream providers of care
- Excessive reliance on clinically and economically inappropriate sites of care
- Lack of coordination in care delivery and lack of an identified regular source of primary care
- Inappropriately high levels of certain types of care
- Indiscriminate and episodic seeking of care (i.e., "doctor shopping")

Taken together, these problems reflect a kind of Medicaid syndrome—restricted access leading to undesirable treatment patterns, which in turn lead to utilization and perhaps quality of care that might be inappropriate or inadequate. The problems interlock and reinforce each other and reflect how difficult it is to modify the system effectively; simply tinkering with payment levels is insufficient.

As noted above, restricted access must be attributed at least in part to the unwillingness of many providers to accept Medicaid payment rates. The result is that care-seeking beneficiaries must find providers who, because of their locations or missions, render care to everyone who presents for care. These providers are commonly either (1) institutional providers such as hospital emergency or outpatient departments, health centers, and clinics located in areas densely populated by low-income individuals or (2) individuals or groups of physicians who by choice or necessity have developed practices that serve Medicaid-eligible populations. The problem is compounded when beneficiaries learn of the willingness of these providers to accept Medicaid payment and thus seek care with the knowledge that they will not be overtly or subtly turned away.

The sheer volume of demand can overload these providers and thus increase the likelihood that the benefits of primary care management will have to be compromised. In addition, structural features of many of the institutional providers, such as hospital emergency departments, make continuity of care problematic since they exist primarily (or exclusively) to render episodic care. Impersonal care invariably results, given the lack of sustained doctor-patient relationships in these settings. A visit is limited to strictly addressing presenting complaints. Amenities are commonly lacking, and long waits followed by brief visits are customary. Referrals might not occur because follow-up tracking is weak, and episodic care is thus perpetuated. Unit records might or might not be maintained, and even when they are available, they are not necessarily consulted.

There are significant adverse economic consequences associated with the undesirable patterns of care described above. The costs of visits to such sites as emergency departments are substantially more than what would be paid for office visits of comparable clinical content (Fleming and Jones 1983). Redundant diagnostic work might be repeated as patients are shuttled (or shuttle themselves) from clinic to clinic or site to site, and records might not adequately reflect previous work performed. Lack of follow-up on referrals might lead to disjointed care that is both ineffective and inefficient. The patient might return to the institution because desired outcomes have not been achieved. Undesirable medical sequelae, such as avoidable hospitalizations, might result if unresolved problems worsen. Waiting time and travel costs can be substantial and are often undervalued because of the nonworking status of most beneficiaries. Furthermore, the dilution of individual provider responsibility in institutional settings can diminish a sense of accountability for resources consumed by patients. In the truest sense, these settings epitomize unmanaged and uncoordinated health care delivery.

It is ironic that a lack of patient care management due to restricted access could lead to higher volumes of care that mask the true limited-access problem. Patients without a regular source of care are more likely to engage in doctor shopping since they do not have available a guide or counselor whose judgment they trust. Moreover, such relationships could avoid unneeded visits for the "worried well." The lack of an identified and familiar source of primary care can, in fact, reduce the tendency to call for advice and reassurance that could avoid the need for emergency department visits that are not medically justified. Uncoordinated care or delayed care can also result in ineffective or deferred treatment that can ultimately mean more services are consumed. Each of these situations may lead to increases in quantity of services rendered without any real contribution to improved health or health status. Yet they are common features of care-seeking behavior for Medicaid beneficiaries.

The Primary Care Management Strategy

Although the absence of primary care management and its consequences, such as diminished access, have long been recognized in Medicaid, the central question has been how to obtain primary care management within the very real financial constraints faced by state programs. Early attempts included promoting the expansion of primary care capacity through the support or establishment of community and neighborhood health centers that functioned as freestanding outpatient departments or emergency rooms (Saward and Greenlick 1972). Often engaging indigenous populations in the design and governance of these programs, these facilities sought to render high volumes of comprehensive services using a broad spectrum of health and social service personnel. Although they focused on serving truly medically indigent patients, in time most programs developed a broader payer mix and grew to rely on multiple sources of financing, including Medicaid. A number of these centers became major players in the emergence of PCCM in the 1980s (Freund et al. 1990).

Another model employed to address the absence of adequate primary care management capacity in Medicaid was the encouragement in the mid-1970s of voluntary enrollment of Medicaid beneficiaries in HMOs (Fuller and Koziol 1977; Gaus, Cooper, and Hirschman 1976). Despite some success on a small scale in selected locations (Luft 1981) and some very notable failures in California due to serious marketing abuses and weak monitoring (Chavin and Treseder 1977), this strategy made little headway. A major reason was that because they were voluntary programs, Medicaid beneficiaries had little to gain by opting into what was a more restrictive and, at the time, rather novel alternative. Although by private indemnity standards the average HMO benefit package seemed a rich one, so was the Medicaid benefit package. Thus the incentive to switch was weak—a problem that persists today for voluntary HMO enrollment programs.

Another major reason for lack of growth was the insufficiency of capitation rates that typically were established from a Medicaid FFS base. Since the loss-ratio measure (capitation premium revenues versus expenditures for services) was the yardstick used to ascertain viability of enrolling a particular group, the use of the low FFS basis virtually assured that established HMOs would have an adverse loss ratio. To balance expenditures with capitation payments would require reductions in utilization that might not be attainable or desirable. Related to this was the concern that Medicaid members might somehow be more difficult to integrate into a prepaid setting that ostensibly promoted prevention and health maintenance, given their tradition of episodic care and poor health habits (Luft 1981). Finally, the intermittent nature of eligibility for public assistance and Medicaid was problematic for PHPs that need predictability in enrollment and in the stream of anticipated capitation revenues.

In an effort to stimulate alternative approaches, states were encouraged to avail themselves of what were, at that time, relatively unknown regulatory waiver opportunities that permitted demonstration programs that might be at variance with a state's Medicaid plan and federal regulations (Galblum and Trieger 1982). The logic of these waivers was to allow new delivery and payment systems to be developed that were both nontraditional in design and not uniformly implemented, as a substitute in selected areas for the traditional full Medicaid program. To allow for experimentation and gradual phase-in of programs, for example, the statewideness requirement to ensure uniform Medicaid programs could be waived. Adaptations of private sector models to accommodate special needs and problems in Medicaid were encouraged, as were approaches that might include elements of competition, reflecting the appeal of Enthoven's (1978) "Consumer Choice Health Plan." Primary care case management, or gatekeeping, initially implemented in the SAFECO United Healthcare Program, was seen as a particularly appealing prototype (Moore 1979; Moore, Martin, and Richardson 1983; Bachman 1982).

The initial wave of demonstration programs included a series of features that were intended to respond to the Medicaid syndrome (NGA 1985; Merlis 1987; Freund and Hurley 1987). In most programs, beneficiaries were required to enroll with a primary care case manager of their choosing, who then would provide care directly or authorize all referral care. The primary care physician (or organization in some cases) performed a gatekeeping function in that beneficiaries were required to contact them before seeking care from other providers. In some programs, risk-sharing schemes were employed to encourage the PCP-gatekeepers to more aggressively manage care. A wide variety of incentive programs was developed in these PCP networks, which paralleled those being introduced in the growing area of independent practice association (IPA-model) HMOs. Finally, several of the early programs embraced the competitive notion that if sufficient providers chose to participate as gatekeepers, beneficiaries would have expanded choice and could select those providers who differentiated themselves based on higher quality or more desirable benefit packages.

It should be emphasized that the explicit goal of these programs—in fact a condition for the approval of their waivers—was demonstrated cost-effectiveness. For two reasons, this goal was broader than simply cost containment. First, access to necessary care could not be impeded by the adopted program design. Second, the principal vehicle for cost containment—PCCM—was expected to control expenditures through improved service coordination and management and not simply through the elimination of care. The rationale for PCCM was that it could offer beneficiaries a qualified, stable source of primary care services that could alter patterns of use that had evolved in an environment of constrained access, and that had resulted in costly and potentially ineffective care. Despite these conditions, critics raised concerns about both threats inherent in the restrictions on freedom of choice and the potential inadequacy of beneficiary safeguards.

Primary Care Case Management: Opportunity or Threat?

Because of the many problems of the Medicaid program, its defenders are few in number. In recent years, as the program has been battered by fiscal crises at the federal and state levels and strained by rapidly rising health care costs, the number of its supporters has shrunk even further. On the other hand, sincere efforts at reform frequently have run afoul of advocacy groups that see the changes only as part of a continuing effort by public agencies to vacate social responsibilities and introduce strategies that simply seek to save money largely with disregard for beneficiaries' welfare. Thus, efforts to salvage some of the undelivered ideals of Medicaid might run counter to new approaches to offer a guarantee of adequate benefits. Because of this, PCCM programs have invoked a surprising amount of trenchant criticism from Medicaid advocates who view it as a serious threat to beneficiaries (Spitz and Abramson 1987; Rosenblatt 1986). Both advocates and reformers seem to be justified to a degree, but both consider themselves to be completely right.

The most controversial feature of PCCM programs is the restriction on full freedom to choose a provider. This restriction means that not only is self-referral to a specialist proscribed behavior, but also essentially all care must be funneled through a single portal of entry or gatekeeper. Critics suggest that this procedure can prevent a beneficiary from getting necessary care if the beneficiary is unable to persuade the gatekeeper to provide the referral. The restriction of true emergency care, however, is prohibited under the federal waivers allowing these programs. While supporters of gatekeeping respond that the restriction on freedom of choice of provider has long been common in HMOs and is currently widespread in private sector managed care, the Medicaid setting might be different. Out-of-plan or out-of-network use in the private sector plans typically means members must pay all or a substantial part of the cost of this uncovered care out-of-pocket. Such unauthorized care for the Medicaid beneficiary who has, by definition, limited financial resources, might be more difficult to acquire. For this reason alone, gatekeeping might have more momentous implications in Medicaid than it does in the private sector.

Given the heightened responsibility of the gatekeeper as the exclusive portal of entry, the selection of physicians and the specification of gatekeeper responsibilities take on special importance. Critics have contended this aspect was notably weak in early gatekeeper programs, where criteria for the selection and monitoring of provider performance were absent or minimal at best. Consequently, they argued, physicians were not fully cognizant of their duties and program developers lacked standards with which to monitor performance. Similar to the SAFECO program (Moore 1979; Moore, Martin, and Richardson 1983), which identified inadequate training of physicians and patients as a problem in gatekeeping, Medicaid programs have also engaged in a substantial amount of learning by doing. To avoid adverse consequences, however, many early programs consciously avoided rigorous enforcement of some gatekeeper requirements, such as obtaining prior authorization for referrals.

Early Medicaid experience with HMO enrollment in California earned notoriety for poor implementation and the exploitation of beneficiaries through shabby enrollment practices (Chavin and Treseder 1977; Rosenblatt 1986). This experience sowed the seeds of skepticism toward any Medicaid initiatives that required beneficiaries to select into systems of care in which their choice of providers would be restricted. The selection or choice-of-plan process was unfamiliar for most beneficiaries and for most public sector program managers (Luft 1981). The choice process crystallized a number of concerns, including (1) adequately informing beneficiaries about their options, (2) avoiding abuses in plan marketing, (3) dealing with persons failing to exercise a choice, (4) handling complaints and decisions to change plans or providers, and (5) monitoring satisfaction and quality of care. Inexperience and unfamiliarity did result in serious problems in these areas, which critics saw as the confirmation of their concerns about whether state Medicaid agencies had the knowledge, ability, and resources to mount these ambitious new initiatives. It was apparent that offering a managed care product carried with it burdens that went beyond those found in the traditional passive-purchaser role of Medicaid.

Not only were there technical problems in understanding and operationalizing gatekeeping adequately for physicians and patients, but also ideological and psychological concerns were raised by skeptics. Despite longstanding use of prepayment or capitation in HMOs, its employment with individual physicians or physician networks in the public sector was troubling to many observers. This skepticism rested on the question, How could a program that was already substantially underpaying providers somehow encourage them to take further financial risks in the hopes of improving their revenues?

The early programs were also inattentive to quality review and assurance (Freund and Hurley 1987). Moreover, where private (HMO) or quasi-public (HIO) intermediaries were prepaid by Medicaid, concern was expressed that this was a deceptive kind of privatization of the program that diluted public responsibility. Additionally, the HIO model presented other concerns, given their limited capital asset base and exemption from the reserve requirements placed on insurers. However, the Consolidated Omnibus Budget Reconciliation Act of 1985 (COBRA) has virtually prohibited the development of new HIOs.

More directly, the use of financial incentives to discourage referral care, or perhaps even primary care, introduced the possibility of a conflict of interest for primary care gatekeepers. These concerns continue to occupy the minds of PCPs and appear in the pages of their professional journals (see, for example, Ellsburg and Stephens 1989). For many Medicaid advocates, conflict of interest was a risk common in the private sector from which they wished to protect beneficiaries. A final concern in the implementation of these programs was the potential disruption of existing doctor-patient relationships for persons who had a prior usual source of care but whose source did not qualify or did not choose to participate as a primary care gatekeeper. In such instances, unfortunately, the introduction of gatekeeping clearly could work at cross-purposes to its goal of promoting continuity of care through primary care management.

Despite these concerns, the growth of Medicaid managed care since the early 1980s has been dramatic. As shown previously in Figure 1.2, the number of enrollees in managed care programs grew more than tenfold during this period. By 1992, there were approximately 3.6 million Medicaid beneficiaries in managed care overall. Of these, 1.5 million were in HMOs, 1.2 million in PCCM programs, and 0.9 million in HIOs/prepaid health plans, up from approximately 270,000 in 1981.

Conclusion

Bringing managed care to Medicaid has proven to be at least as challenging as it has been in the private sector. The reasons for this can be found in the history of the program and the evolution of a delivery system for Medicaid that has manifest shortcomings and that has proven highly intractable to reform. The absence of obvious alternatives has resulted in the encouragement of a wide assortment of approaches that fall under the general rubric of PCCM. Foremost among the features of these programs is the attempt to make primary care management available to persons for whom its potential benefits are substantial.

These programs have taken many different forms, as described in the next chapter. This variety affords an opportunity to compare differing structures and designs to determine whether they differ on outcomes. Moreover, given the many critics of these programs, it is essential to know whether one or more approaches can achieve desired outcomes while minimizing risks or providing adequate safeguards to beneficiaries against these risks. Finally, assessing the array of existing programs allows informed speculation about what the next generation of Medicaid managed care will look like.

References

Bachman, S. 1982. *Case Management as a Cost Effective Approach to Improving Health Services to Medicaid Beneficiaries.* Grant No. 11-P-90666. Baltimore, MD: Office of Research and Demonstrations, HCFA.

Chavin, D., and A. Treseder. 1977. "California's Prepaid Health Plans." *Hastings Law Journal* 28: 685–760.

Cohen, W. 1985. "Reflections on the Enactment of Medicare and Medicaid." *Health Care Financing Review* (Annual Supplement): 3–11.

Cromwell, J., and J. Mitchell. 1984. "An Economic Model of Large Medicaid Practices." *Health Services Research* 19(2): 197–218.

Davidson, S., J. Cromwell, and R. Schurman. 1986. "Medicaid Myths: Trends in Medicaid Expenditures and the Prospects for Reform." *Journal of Health Politics, Policy and Law* 10(4): 699–726.

Ellsburg, K., and G. Stephens. 1989. "Can the Family Physician Avoid Conflict of Interest in the Gatekeeper Role?" *Journal of Family Practice* 28: 698–704.

Enthoven, A. 1978. "Consumer-Choice Health Plan." *New England Journal of Medicine* 298(12): 650–58.

Fleming, N., and H. Jones. 1983. "The Impact of Outpatient Department and Emergency Room Use on Costs in the Texas Medicaid Program." *Medical Care* 21(9): 892–910.

Freund, D. 1984. *Medicaid Reform: Four Studies of Case Management.* Washington, DC: American Enterprise Institute.

Freund, D., and R. Hurley. 1987. "Managed Care in Medicaid: Selected Issues in Program Origins, Design, and Research." *Annual Review of Public Health* 8: 137–63.

Freund, D., R. Hurley, K. Adamache, and J. Mauskopf. 1990. "The Performance of Urban and Public Hospitals and NHCs Under Medicaid Capitation Programs." *Hospital & Health Services Administration* 35(4): 525–46.

Fuller, N., and K. Koziol. 1977. "Medicaid Utilization in a Prepaid Group Practice Health Plan." *Medical Care* 15(9): 705–37.

Galblum, T., and S. Trieger. 1982. "Demonstrations of Alternative Delivery Systems Under Medicare and Medicaid." *Health Care Financing Review* 3(1): 1–12.

Gaus, C., B. Cooper, and C. Hirschman. 1976. "Contrast Between HMO and FFS Performance." *Social Security Bulletin* 39(5): 3–14.

Hurley, R., and D. Freund. 1988. *Utilization Management: Perspectives from the Medicaid Program.* Background paper prepared for the Institute of Medicine Committee on Utilization Management. Washington, DC: National Academy of Sciences, Institute of Medicine.

Luft, H. 1981. *HMOs: Dimensions of Performance.* New York: John Wiley & Sons.

Merlis, M. 1987. *Medicaid Contracts with HMOs and Prepaid Health Plans.* Washington, DC: National Governors' Association.

Mitchell, J., and J. Cromwell. 1980. "Medicaid Mills: Fact or Fiction." *Health Care Financing Review* 2(4): 37–49.

Moore, S. 1979. "Cost Containment Through Risk-Sharing by Primary Care Physicians." *New England Journal of Medicine* 300(24): 1359–62.

Moore, S., D. Martin, and W. Richardson. 1983. "Does the Primary Care Gatekeeper Control the Costs of Health Care? Lessons from the SAFECO Experience." *New England Journal of Medicine* 309(22): 1400–04.

National Governors' Association (NGA). 1985. *Prepaid and Managed Care Under Medicaid: Overview of Current Initiatives.* Washington: The Association.

Perloff, J., P. Kletke, and K. Neckerman. 1987. *Medicaid and Pediatric Primary Care.* Baltimore: Johns Hopkins University Press.

Reinhardt, U. 1985. "Comments on 20 Years of Medicare and Medicaid." *Health Care Financing Review* (Annual Supplement): 105–11.

Rosenblatt, R. 1986. "Medicaid Primary Care Case Management: The Doctor-Patient Relationship and the Politics of Privatization." *Case Western Reserve University Law Review* 36: 915.

Saward, E. W., and M. R. Greenlick. 1972. "Health Policy and the HMO." *Milbank Memorial Fund Quarterly* 50(2): 147–76.

Sloan, F., J. Mitchell, and J. Cromwell. 1978. "Physician Participation in State Medicaid Programs." *Journal of Human Resources* 18(Supplement): 211–46.

Spitz, B., and J. Abramson. 1987. "Competition, Capitation, and Case Management: Barriers to Strategic Reform." *Milbank Memorial Fund Quarterly* 65(3): 348–68.

Chapter 4

Describing and Classifying Programs

Many different approaches to PCCM have been adopted to address the dual goals of improving cost-effectiveness and enhancing access to health care for Medicaid beneficiaries. In part the variation is due to the explicit encouragement of variation in the federal regulations. The variation is also due to a lack of evidence to guide program developers who have therefore had to apply their own ingenuity in program design. Resource constraints on state Medicaid agencies have also played a role in determining both the desirable and the possible. Finally, local health care market conditions represent an additional and significant set of external factors for defining which program designs are considered in principle and which ones are implemented in practice.

The first decade of PCCM resulted in the production of an enormous amount of descriptive information on program design and development. Beginning with Freund (1984) and continuing through the MCD Evaluation (RTI 1989), the MPE (ORD 1987), the Arizona AHCCCS evaluation (SRI International 1989), and numerous monographs by the NGA (e.g., NGA 1985), a huge volume of case studies was produced. These studies, in aggregate, present a useful overview of the varied approaches adopted by these programs, detailing policy and program strategies at the local and state levels to respond to the problems discussed in Chapter 3. The case studies are portraits of public agencies challenged by the complexity of managed care program development and often encountering resistance from providers, beneficiaries, and other interest groups.

In some respects, however, these case studies have impeded a broader understanding of the Medicaid PCCM phenomenon because they have served to highlight the differences and idiosyncracies of these diverse initiatives. This situation is not surprising since the programs that have been launched typically are a product of mutual adjustment and structuring based on beneficiary needs, program developer goals, resource availability, acceptability to key constituencies, and the delicate and normally prolonged negotiation leading up to implementation. Thus, focusing closely on the particulars of each program would suggest that they defy generalization. Added to this has been the absence, until recently, of systematically analyzed impact data from these programs. This lack of data has prevented researchers from drawing conclusions regarding patterns of effects associated with the varied program designs.

However, the amount of available evidence regarding program effects has increased substantially during the past three years. Given these findings, it is important to examine and classify program designs to enable policymakers, analysts, and researchers to build a systematic body of knowledge on PCCM in the Medicaid context.

We collected detailed program descriptions and related reports on 25 PCCM programs for the purposes of this study; a systematic summary of each of the reviewed programs is contained in the appendix at the end of this book. These programs were selected because of the availability of analytical evidence. In some cases the data and analyses were part of a program waiver renewal application; for others independent evaluations had been prepared assessing program impact.

Overall, more than 1.2 million Medicaid beneficiaries have been enrolled in PCCM programs. This book provides the most extensive and exhaustive cataloguing of programs to date; however, because documentation on the many other programs and initiatives is sparse or of poor quality, this book is still incomplete with regard to some ways states have attempted to bring primary care management to Medicaid beneficiaries. Nonetheless, the picture is potentially highly informative if we draw out of the years of experience (and volumes of narrative) some general patterns from well-substantiated efforts relating to PCCM program design and implementation.

Variation in program design alone is addressed in this chapter because program design is assumed to be fundamentally and directly related to program outcomes. In practice, of course, program implementation also has an important bearing on program outcomes. However, we need an established baseline of comparison on structure before we can examine variations in implementation.

Toward a Typology of Medicaid Managed Care

The development of classification schemes is a challenging but essential enterprise in all scientific endeavors. Classification schemes are necessary for identifying patterns and establishing program context; in addition, they also allow improved communication and the transmittal of accumulated evidence. When classification schemes are missing, inadequate, or outmoded because of changes in the phenomenon being studied, confusion is created or heightened. A current example in the health care field is the diminishing usefulness of the traditional classification of HMOs (Welch, Hillman, and Pauly 1990). The goal of efforts to revise HMO classification schemes, and the goal of classification schemes in general, is to identify features that capture the sources and range of variation on important dimensions of the system being observed.

Identifying key features useful for distinguishing among PCCM programs in Medicaid begins by examining the many ways in which the programs differ, based on a review of the large volume of case study material. Ideally, these features should be related to program outcomes, and their relative importance should be empirically validated as producing differential program effects. It is also desirable for the detailed features to be configured or synthesized into a limited number of program prototypes. These prototypes can then be used to categorize similar programs and to allow program findings to be synthesized and compared across program prototypes.

Initial efforts at developing classification schemes for PCCM programs were made by the NGA in 1985 (NGA 1985). These approaches focused on (1) whether capitation or prepayment was used, (2) what type provider system was being employed, (3) the administrative structure of the programs, (4) the mandatory or voluntary nature of the program, and (5) the eligible groups being enrolled. These features were generally specified, but the full range of variation was not detailed. Moreover, the asymmetrical nature of the program designs (i.e., who administered them, whether capitation payments were made to providers or to risk-assuming intermediaries, what the range of case manager responsibilities was, etc.) was not well-captured in the NGA descriptive classifications. As programs increased in number and variation, the classification had to be modified to accommodate and depict them.

In 1988, Hurley and Freund published a typology for Medicaid PCCM programs (Hurley and Freund 1988) that incorporated and expanded on the earlier classifications, including one developed by Hurley (1986) as part of an overview of the MCDs. Hurley and Freund identified six significant design features on which programs differed: (1) enrollment, (2) organizational approach, (3) case manager qualifications and selection, (4) case manager service range responsibility, (5) case manager payment method, and (6) responsibility for determining payment methods to other program providers. The typology also specified the range of variation observed for each feature, as summarized in Table 4.1. Finally, the article illustrated how the typology could be used to identify similarities and differences among a representative group of programs. However, because the classification

Table 4.1 A Typology of Medicaid Case Management Programs

Type of Recipient Enrollment	*Organizational Approach*	*Case Manager Participation*	*Case Manager Service Range Responsibility*	*Case Manager Payment Method*	*Payment Method for Other Providers*
1. Voluntary	1. Contract with risk-assuming intermediary that subcontracts with case managers	1. Limited to primary care provider	1. Primary care provision with specified brokering/ authorizing duties	1. FFS	1. Traditional Medicaid
2. Mandatory	2. Direct Medicaid agency contracts with case managers	2. Limited to primary care organizations	2. Provision or arrangement of virtually all Medicaid services	2. FFS with case manager fee	2. Negotiated by risk-assuming intermediary
		3. Limited to prepaid health plans		3. FFS with shared savings opportunities	3. Negotiated by case manager
				4. Capitation with shared-saving opportunities	
				5. Capitation	

Source: Hurley and Freund 1988.

scheme was not extended to synthesize a set of program aggregates or to identify specific program prototypes, it has served more as a set of classification rules than as a policy-relevant tool. The authors concluded that the real utility of this typology would be when a sufficiently large number of programs could be classified and findings from them reported on an aggregated basis. Thus, the 1988 typology led directly to the current study, which both applies the classification approach and attempts to validate its usefulness in PCCM program differentiation. Appendix 4.1 provides definitions and logic relating to each of the key features of the typology.

Employing the Typology to Classify Programs

Appendix 4.2 presents the classification of the 25 programs described in the appendix at the end of the book, using the Hurley and Freund (1988) typology. Appendix 4.2 also serves as a summary of the selected programs. Although this set of programs might not necessarily be representative of the universe of PCCM programs, it does demonstrate that the typology is effective for classification purposes and that the range of variation proposed in the typology is manifested across these 25 programs. Table 4.2 summarizes the distribution of programs on each feature of the typology.

The implications of the classification for specific elements of the typology are discussed below.

Enrollment

Of the 25 programs examined, 19 of them were mandatory while 6 were voluntary. There are several reasons for the relatively limited number of voluntary programs represented. The first reason is that voluntary programs that enroll Medicaid beneficiaries in HMOs are not required to obtain federal waivers (which require independent evaluations); thus, less documentation is typically available for these programs. Second, as mentioned earlier, these programs are widely acknowledged as attracting disappointing enrollment. They have therefore waned in their appeal because the level of effort to initiate them has frequently failed to yield commensurate dividends. A third more technical reason is that programs that permit voluntary enrollment are subject to selection bias (i.e., nonrandom enrollment patterns) that can mask true program effects. For example, apparently lower cost and use could be due primarily to healthier persons enrolling in a voluntary program instead of due to any specific PCCM effect. This issue is evident in some of the program results, although with the exception of a recent RAND study (Buchanan et al. 1992), few analyses have systematically tested for selection bias in voluntary programs. Finally,

Table 4.2 Program Summary by Attributes

Attribute	*Number of Programs*
Type of enrollment	
Voluntary	6
Mandatory	19
Organizational approach	
HIO/intermediary	7
State-administered	18
Case manager participation	
Primary care providers	7
Primary care providers and primary care organizations	7
Primary care organizations only	5
Prepaid health plans	6
Case manager responsibility	
Providing/brokering/authorizing	19
Full scope of services	6
Case manager payment methods	
FFS	2
FFS with case manager fee	5
FFS with shared savings	1
Capitation with shared savings	11
Capitation	6
Payment methods for other providers	
Medicaid payment schedule	13
Negotiated by HIO	6
Negotiated by HMO	6

the major analytical studies—the MCD Evaluation and the MPE—each had access to only one voluntary program among the dozen programs they examined overall.

Organizational approach

The organizational approaches adopted also broadly reflect two major design variations, with 18 programs administered by state Medicaid agencies or the local surrogates and 7 programs operated by HIOs under contract with the state agencies. Three of the HIOs were in California; one is no longer in operation. In addition, the HIO in Kentucky was discontinued several years ago. The Washington State and Itasca County (Minnesota) programs are of note as they are predominantly rural sites that have adopted the HIO model. HealthPASS in Philadelphia is the only urban-based HIO in the study. It was mentioned earlier that since the COBRA legislation of 1985, Congress has virtually prohibited the establishment of additional HIOs. Those HIOs that continue are in effect grandfathered in as they continue operation.

The other consistent feature inherent with the HIO organizational model is that in every case the state agencies have virtually guaranteed that there will be some savings associated with the HIO contracts. They do so by paying a capitation rate per beneficiary that is discounted from expected FFS expenditures, leaving the HIO with the risk of actual expenditures for patient care. This issue is discussed further in Chapter 7.

The characterization of an HIO as an organizational approach to PCCM rather than as a special case of state contracting with a PHP variant can be disputed. The basis for this decision is that while the HIO is a risk-assuming intermediary, it is not a preexisting integrated delivery system such as that found in HMOs. In essence, the state agency subcontracts administration to these entities and charges them with the development of a provider network and the full range of enrollment and management responsibilities for covered beneficiaries. When the original PCCM typology was developed, the authors noted that it was essential to be able to examine separately any programs that had very distinct delivery systems, such as those developed in the early California programs (Hurley and Freund 1988). Adding the method-of-payment feature permitted this to be done. In contemporary terms, the HIO functions like a carrier-sponsored PPO, which is acknowledged by most observers to be qualitatively different from a PHP or an HMO.

Among the state-administered programs, not all are statewide, therefore requiring a federal waiver from the requirement of statewide program uniformity. Two programs were statewide by design and from inception, while four others are moving toward statewide implementation incrementally, although they might never fully reach this goal because of limited provider participation in rural counties. The voluntary program in New Jersey was to be implemented statewide but never achieved this status prior to its evolution into a state-sponsored HMO, the Garden State Health Plan. Several states have targeted their programs both initially and over time to urban areas, which typically have high Medicaid beneficiary concentrations. Only one state (Minnesota) has both urban and rural components in its design.

Case manager qualifications and selection

A total of seven programs have restricted primary care gatekeepers to individual PCPs or groups. Primary care physicians typically include general practitioners, family practice physicians, pediatricians, general internists, and obstetricians-gynecologists (OB-GYNs) to the extent they can provide the full range of primary care services. These programs explicitly mandate a link between an individual physician and a beneficiary to take advantage of the benefits of primary care management via gatekeeping. In virtually every one of these programs an implicit goal is to permit beneficiaries to have their prior usual sources of care become their gatekeepers. This requirement has meant that most of the programs have continued to use FFS as the method of payment.

There are also seven programs that permit primary care organizations as well as individual PCPs to enroll beneficiaries. These organizations are usually public or private health clinics or hospital outpatient departments in the program area.

Another five programs engage only large groups of physicians, such as hospitals or university-affiliated group practices, or specifically identified health clinics. Three other programs require physicians to form or join risk pools to participate, although beneficiaries are still enrolled with individual physicians. The remaining programs contract exclusively with PHPs. These plans may be preexisting HMOs, new organizations structured to perform as HMOs, or quasi-HMOs such as neighborhood health clinics and hospital outpatient departments functioning under prepayment and fully at risk. We use the term "PHP" to represent more generic models of organizations receiving prepayment for a full range of services. Some PHPs are licensed entities that qualify as HMOs. For the purpose of the typology, we use PHP and HMO interchangeably since the distinction is not a critical factor.

Service range responsibility

The case management responsibility in 19 of the programs is specified as providing primary care services and brokering, referring, or authorizing all referral services. The other 6 programs of the 25 require participating case managers to assume full responsibility for all services, since in virtually every case the providers are PHPs with a fully developed provider network. However, there are some minor differences in how the programs specify directly provided services. These differences are related to the scope of services for which case managers are paid. For example, several programs pay case managers to provide routine laboratory and x-ray work or to make attending physician visits during hospital stays. In effect, this requirement defines these services as *primary care* (i.e., services expected to be provided by the primary care case manager). On the other hand, all the programs require emergency department use to be preauthorized, unless the event is a bona fide emergency. Likewise, care provided by specialists is required to be authorized by the case manager. The plans typically verify the case manager's authorization of specialty care before specialty care claims are paid.

The programs that assign full-service responsibility to the case-managing organization itself might be qualitatively different for a basic reason: the techniques of care management, including primary care gatekeeping, are left to the discretion of the PHP managers instead of to the providers. Some of these plans, such as IPA-model HMOs, use a gatekeeping approach similar to that used in the 19 programs just described. Others do not do so for either structural, managerial, or philosophical reasons. In such cases, the organization itself is performing case management, including monitoring utilization and maintaining 24-hour accessibility. To date there are no studies that contrast the performance of these arrangements with the performance of HMOs that have an individualized PCCM focus.

Case manager payment method

Fee-for-service payment has been the method of choice in most programs requiring gatekeepers to be individual PCPs. Two programs pay only FFS while another five also pay a nominal case management fee of approximately $1.50 to $3 per enrollee per month. One program permits FFS-paid PCPs to share in savings resulting from reduced referral care, which in effect means the case manager fee or augmentation is a variable amount usually subject to some ceiling.

Eleven of the programs place PCPs at some financial risk by paying them a capitation amount. This rate is actuarially computed to cover the cost of care for the average enrollee for the services for which the case manager is responsible. Case managers are also permitted in some programs to participate in residuals in either individual or pooled referral accounts. The range of variation in these arrangements is substantial and often very complex. The complexity results from behavioral assumptions that program developers have about how best to intensify the pressures on gatekeepers to manage care rigorously. In some cases, straight division of savings or losses in referral accounts between physicians and Medicaid programs is used. In others, more involved formulas have been developed to discourage some behaviors and encourage others. A refined assessment of differences among these methods requires detailed actuarial studies beyond the scope of normally available data.

Within the 11 programs that put the case manager at some financial risk, there is an important distinction not explicitly incorporated into the typology in its current form. Several programs either (1) pay capitation only to groups or pools of PCPs or (2) pool the expenses debited to referral accounts to dilute the direct impact of risk-sharing on individual physicians. Others have chosen not to employ either of these strategies but instead have set stop-loss ceilings on the basis of individual beneficiaries or individual physician panels. Thus, in the former program types there are two tiers through which the risk-sharing is filtered. There is only one tier in the latter type. This issue is also raised in Welch, Hillman, and Pauly's (1990) proposed taxonomy for HMOs and is used to differentiate among different types of HMOs. The remaining programs, most of which use HMOs exclusively as service delivery providers, rely on a single capitation payment. The organization then allocates this payment to meet service delivery responsibilities for which it is contractually obligated.

Methods for paying other providers

The variation on this feature shows 13 programs paying other providers via traditional Medicaid payment methods; in 6 programs, payment methods are subject to negotiation between the physician case manager and the network or panel members, including hospitals; and in the remaining programs, HIO-negotiated payment arrangements with other service providers are used. The accumulated evidence indicates that this feature of the typology is adequately subsumed in the information regarding organizational approach and case manager selection and therefore is largely a redundant category.

Synthesizing Program Design Features into Prototypes

The classification system employed in the Hurley and Freund (1988) typology allows for many possible combinations of program designs. Most of these designs have not been attempted and thus there is no experience to report from them. Many cells in the hypothetical full typology would also have only one or two programs in them, and some possible combinations reflect infeasible designs. These points highlight the limitation of a classification system that is not sufficiently elaborated to allow the experience of a number of broadly similar programs to be combined.

However, this problem can be addressed by proposing a limited set of program prototypes that combine programs with similar configurations based on the design classification features described in the previous section. Although only a few pure manifestations of each prototype may exist, the objective is to create groups that represent clusters with more similarities than differences in design features. In essence, the prototypes represent a synthesis of program features on which similar programs can be classified. Although the typology allows other configurations to be produced by focusing on features other than how primary care case managers are paid, this dimension is felt to be the most critical and is the basis for the following three program prototypes:

Type 1: FFS primary care gatekeeper enrollment

Type 2: Risk-sharing primary care gatekeeper enrollment

Type 3: HMO or PHP enrollment

Each of the prototypes is described in general terms below and illustrated in Figure 4.1.

Type 1: Fee-for-service primary care gatekeeper enrollment

This model is one of the most common and least intrusive PCCM interventions. Under this arrangement, state agencies or independent HIOs contract with PCPs or PCOs to provide, refer (broker), and authorize virtually all covered services to enrolled beneficiaries. The referring-brokering-authorizing role reflects the expectation that the service responsibility of this provider will be limited to primary care. The primary care gatekeeper is paid FFS for services directly provided and is typically paid a nominal

Figure 4.1 Primary Care Case Management Prototypes

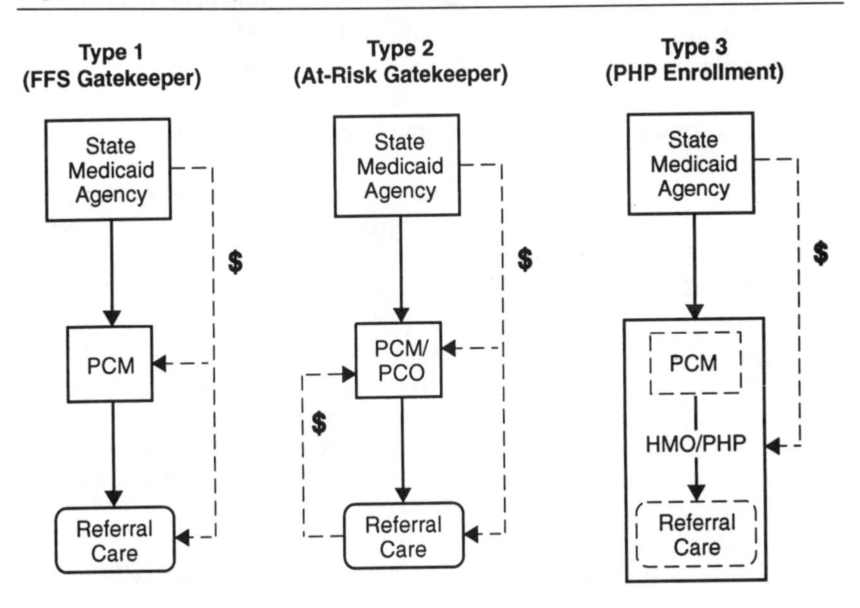

monthly case management fee per enrollee to compensate for administrative responsibilities and expanded availability. Payment methods to other providers rendering gatekeeper-authorized services are determined by the state agency or HIO. Gatekeepers' compensation is unaffected by the referral use experience of their enrollees. The intensity of the intervention is characteristically low, causing minimal disruption to existing practice and referral patterns. The intervention is often selected to maximize provider participation and minimize both provider and beneficiary resistance. Administrative costs are normally lower as well because changes in the basic FFS payment mechanism are limited (RTI 1988).

These programs essentially attempt to extend to beneficiaries the benefits of a regular source of primary care and then to exploit this relationship by encouraging gatekeepers to be judicious managers of services without direct financial incentives. These programs are typically mandatory, with exclusions for special groups and special circumstances. Exclusions are made in part because it is difficult to induce beneficiaries to accept voluntarily the freedom-of-choice restriction of gatekeeping. The intervention is primarily structural and does not contain explicit economic incentives. The exclusive gatekeeper role of an FFS PCP, however, may provide some individual incentive for the substitution of FFS primary care for specialty and nonurgent emergency department care.

Type 2: Risk-sharing primary care gatekeeper enrollment

This model is similar to Type 1, with the principal difference being the method of gatekeeper payment. The range of responsibilities is the same and entities eligible to be gatekeepers are comparable. Likewise, programs can be directly state-administered or HIO-operated. The distinction between Type 1 and Type 2 lies in whether financial incentives in the form of program losses or gains are shared with the gatekeeper. Risk-sharing takes one of two forms: (1) capitation payment for primary care services or (2) sharing in losses or gains in referral service accounts. In most instances, the payment methods for referral providers follow traditional patterns, so losses or gains in such accounts are solely the result of utilization experience rather than altered rates of payment.

These programs couple financial incentives and risk-sharing with the structural features of gatekeeping. Restrictions on beneficiary self-referrals and the substitution of less-costly services are expected to be the major vehicles for savings. As with Type 1 programs, issues regarding state versus HIO administration are relevant primarily regarding administrative costs and the adequacy of funds available to induce providers to participate. One potential advantage of HIO administration is that it allows these entities to negotiate alternative fee arrangements with referral providers, which can improve the cost experience of referral fund accounts. Most of these programs are mandatory for the reason described for Type 1 models.

Type 3: Health maintenance organization or prepaid health plan enrollment

In Type 3 programs, beneficiaries are enrolled with existing HMOs, PHPs, or other institutional providers with the capacity to assume responsibility for the provision of all covered services. Enrollment might be either voluntary or mandatory. A contract might be negotiated directly between the state agency and the plan or between the plan and a risk-assuming intermediary such as an HIO. The plan assumes responsibility for case management and the provision of all covered services in return for a capitation payment. Payment rates for other providers are negotiated by the HMO or PHP.

The assumption of full responsibility for all covered services and the acceptance of a corresponding capitation payment distinguishes Type 3 programs from the other prototypes. Whether a program is voluntary or mandatory has both participation and analytical implications (e.g., selection bias) but presumably would not alter the impact of the program on cost and use for enrollees. The distinction between direct management by the state versus HIO contracting has some administrative as well as risk-sharing implications but again should not alter the expected impact on cost and use. A particularly interesting issue is whether institutional or organizational case management has effects comparable to individual physician case management in the two other prototypes discussed above. Another question, which cannot be answered with data currently available, is whether or not newly created PHPs (e.g., hospital outpatient clinics and neighborhood health centers) perform similarly to the preexisting HMOs or PHPs that choose to participate.

Exhibit 4.1 illustrates how the 25 programs included in this study fit into the three prototypes. The fit in Type 1 and Type 3 is straightforward. Type 2 programs are somewhat more heterogeneous; some programs use a two-tiered risk-sharing approach for case manager compensation while other programs place individual physicians at direct risk and use stop-loss provisions to cushion possible adverse impacts. There are some important administrative differences between these two groups, including the use of risk-sharing pools as a vehicle to calculate and distribute shared gains and losses. This additional administrative effort can be used as a strategy to engage individual physicians as gatekeepers who otherwise would not participate because of real or perceived financial risks.

Despite these arguments, we did not subdivide the Type 2 prototype on the basis of risk-sharing approaches. We made this choice both in the

Exhibit 4.1 Programs Classified by Prototype

Type 1: FFS Gatekeeper
Monterey County (CA) Health Initiative
Colorado Primary Care Physician Program
Kansas Primary Care Network
Kentucky Patient Access and Care System
Michigan Medicaid Physician Sponsor Plan
Minnesota Prepaid Medicaid Demonstration in Itasca County
Missouri Physician Sponsor Plan
Utah's Choice of Health Care Delivery Programs

Type 2: At-Risk Gatekeeper
Health Plan of San Mateo County (CA)*
Santa Barbara County (CA) Health Initiative
Louisville (KY) Citicare Program
Michigan Medicaid Capitated Clinic Plan
Nevada Enrolled Health Plan*
New Jersey Medicaid Personal Physician Plan
Erie County (NY) Physician Case Management Program (Children)*
Children's Medicaid Program of Suffolk County (NY)†
Oregon Medicaid Physician Care Organization Program*
HealthPASS of Philadelphia (PA)
Kitsap (WA) Sound Care Plan*

Type 3: PHP/HMO Enrollment
Arizona Health Care Cost Containment System
Minnesota Prepaid Demonstration Project in Hennepin and Dakota Counties
Missouri Prepaid Health Plan Program
Dayton (OH) Area Health Plan
Washington Voluntary HMO Enrollment in Group Health Cooperative
Wisconsin HMO Program

* These programs have a two-tiered system of risk sharing with physician group or pooling used between payer and primary care gatekeeper.

† Suffolk introduced both augmented FFS and capitation with two groups of primary care gatekeepers but is classified as a Type Two program because of its focus on the effects of prepayment.

interest of parsimony and because it is not yet clear that the two-tiered effect is a design feature with significant implications for program outcomes. After evaluating the evidence of program effects in the next chapter, we discuss further the experience of Type 2 programs regarding detectable patterns of difference between the possible subgroups.

By classifying the programs on individual design features and then configuring these features to create prototypes into which the programs are clustered, we were able to systematically examine program outcomes. Moreover, the outcomes from the programs can still be assessed along individual design features, such as accumulated cost and use experience for voluntary versus mandatory programs. A similar approach can be used to compare program prototypes by contrasting, for example, Type 1 with Type 2 programs on cost and utilization impacts. The comparisons in the next chapter are exploratory and descriptive because the total sample size of 25 is not sufficient to apply statistical tests as would be the case if a larger-scale meta-analysis were possible. However, even the exploratory analysis can serve as an initial comprehensive assessment of Medicaid PCCM.

Appendix 4.1 Definition and Logic of Key Features in Medicaid Case Management Program Typology

Table 4.1 summarized the Medicaid managed care typology developed by Hurley and Freund (1988). The following sections expand on the logic of each of its key features.

Enrollment. Medicaid agencies have to make an initial decision on whether the PCCM program will supplant traditional FFS Medicaid, and thus be a mandatory enrollment program, or whether it will simply be a voluntary enrollment alternative to the traditional FFS program. Given the persistent problem of inducing beneficiaries to enter into a choice-restricting program without having to enrich an already-rich benefit package, voluntary programs have suffered from low enrollment and consistently underperformed expectations for aggregate cost savings. Also, voluntary programs create the possibility of preferred or biased enrollment (biased selection) of lower-cost beneficiaries, thereby reducing potential cost savings.

Organizational approach. The basic choice Medicaid agencies have faced on this dimension is whether the state agency or its local public counterpart, such as a county department of social services, administers the program directly or whether the state contracts with a risk-assuming intermediary or HIO to design and manage the program. There are several important implications of this decision. First, by contracting to pay a capitation rate to the HIO, the state can be assured of savings simply by paying a discount from an estimated FFS basis, irrespective of how beneficiary use and cost experience is affected by the case management program design. Second, decisions regarding program design rest with the HIO, which becomes, essentially, a locally based mini-Medicaid agency—a point some critics have characterized as privatization of Medicaid since these HIOs typically are quasi-public authorities. The characterization of the HIO as a feature of administration rather than of service delivery is among the most controversial aspects of the typology.

Case manager qualification and selection. The decision about what types of providers can qualify as primary care gatekeepers or case managers is lodged with either the state agency or the HIO. The range of variation extends from individuals and groups of PCPs to primary care organizations such as clinics or outpatient departments. Some programs permit both types of providers to participate. Still others have used PHPs, which may be preexisting HMOs or ad hoc plans organized for the purposes of the program. In these cases, the organizations themselves serve as case managers. We use the term "PHP" to represent more generic models of organizations receiving prepayment for a full range of services. Some PHPs are licensed entities that qualify as HMOs. For the purpose of the typology, we use PHP and HMO interchangeably since the distinction is not a critical factor. The selection of case managers is closely linked to the range of service responsibilities and methods of payment for the case managers.

Service range responsibility. Case managers at a minimum formally assume responsibility for performing PCCM. In essence, this means they must have the capacity to provide all primary care services directly and to broker or refer all other care, including the formal preauthorization of referrals and consultations by other providers. (Emergency care for true emergencies is exempted by federal regulations from any preauthorization restrictions.) For providers who are part of organizations that have full-service capacity (i.e., HMOs, PHPs, or other networks of providers), the scope of service responsibility typically extends to all Medicaid-covered services. Thus, the brokering or authorization responsibility is governed by the internal policies of the plan. In some cases the assumption of true primary care gatekeeping might not be met at the individual physician level. In effect, the organization as an entity is responsible for gatekeeping.

Case manager payment methods. Great variation on this feature has been observed among PCCM programs. This variation is directly attributable to the assumptions program managers and developers have made about how to induce or encourage case managers to rigorously perform their gatekeeping function. The variation ranges from continuing to pay FFS and FFS with a case manager fee or other augmentation to a wide assortment of incentive payment systems. A common approach is to pay a capitation for primary care services to gatekeepers or case managers and also to permit them to share in the residuals in referral accounts that can result from reduced utilization due to gatekeepers performing effective utilization management. Some programs have used this approach while still paying case managers on an FFS basis. Finally, capitation for the full scope of services is paid to HMOs and PHPs commensurate with the responsibility they assume for managing the full range of covered services. In a number of the incentive- or capitation-based programs, withhold schemes like those found in IPA-model HMOs are also used to guard against exhausting referral accounts.

Payments to other providers. The responsibility for determining the methods and amounts of payments to providers who are not case managers, including hospitals and specialists, also varies within these programs. Three general approaches have been observed. The first is to continue to pay these providers under prevailing Medicaid arrangements. The second is to allow the capitated HMOs/PHPs to negotiate payment methods directly with other providers who are part of their panel or provider network. Finally, in sites where the program is under the jurisdiction of the contracting HIO, decisions about how to pay other providers may reside with the intermediary, which must make all payments out of the capitation amounts the Medicaid agency pays it. In practice, then, this feature is largely determined by the organizational approach adopted and whether PHPs are the case managers.

Appendix 4.2 Primary Care Case Management Programs: Structural Characteristics and Design Features

Program	*Date Established*	*Maximum Number Enrolled*	*Enrollment*	*Organizational Approach*
Arizona Health Care Cost Containment System (AHCCCS)	1982	226,000	Mandatory	State
Monterey County (CA) Health Initiative	1983	22,000	Mandatory	HIO
Health Plan of San Mateo (CA)	1987	31,000	Mandatory	HIO
Santa Barbara (CA) Health Initiative	1983	25,000	Mandatory	HIO
Colorado Primary Care Physician Program (PCPP)	1982	72,000	Mandatory	State
Kansas Primary Care Network	1984	78,000	Mandatory	State
Kentucky Patient Access and Care (KenPAC) System	1986	195,000	Mandatory	State
Citicare (Louisville, KY)	1982	40,000	Mandatory	State
Michigan Medicaid Capitated Clinic Plan	1983	9,000	Voluntary	State
Michigan Medicaid Physician Sponsor Plan	1982	160,000	Voluntary/	State
Minnesota Prepaid Demonstration in Hennepin and Dakota Counties	1986	24,000	Mandatory	State

Case Manager Selection	*Service Range Responsibility*	*Case Manager Payment Method*	*Other Provider Payment*
PCP/PCO	Full	Capitation	Negotiated by case manager
PCP/PCO	P/B/A	FFS+	Negotiated by HIO
PCP/PCO	P/B/A	Capitation/SSO	Negotiated by HIO
PCP/PCO	P/B/A	Capitation/SSO	Negotiated by HIO
PCP	P/B/A	FFS/SSO	Traditional
PCP	P/B/A	FFS+	Traditional
PCP/PCO	P/B/A	FFS+	Traditional
PCP/PCO	P/B/A	Capitation/SSO	Traditional
PCO	P/B/A	Capitation/SSO	Traditional
PCP	P/B/A	FFS+	Traditional
PHP	Full	Capitation	Negotiated by case manager

Continued

Appendix 4.2 Continued

Program	*Date Established*	*Maximum Number Enrolled*	*Enrollment*	*Organizational Approach*
Minnesota Prepaid Demonstration in Itasca County	1985	3,400	Mandatory	HIO
Missouri Physician Sponsor Plan	1983	4,000	Mandatory	State
Missouri Prepaid Health Plan Program	1983	12,000	Mandatory	State
Nevada Enrolled Health Plan	1983	4,000	Voluntary	State
New Jersey Medicaid Personal Physician Plan	1984	12,000	Voluntary	State
Erie County (NY) Physician Case Management Program (Children)	1987	1,166	Voluntary	State
Children's Medicaid Program, Suffolk County, NY	1983	4,000	Voluntary	State
Dayton (OH) Area Health Plan	1989	40,000	Mandatory	State
Oregon Medicaid Physician Care Organization Program	1984	53,000	Mandatory	State
HealthPASS Philadelphia, PA	1986	87,000	Mandatory	HIO

Case Manager Selection	*Service Range Responsibility*	*Case Manager Payment Method*	*Other Provider Payment*
PCP	P/B/A	FFS/SSO	Negotiated by HIO
PCP	P/B/A	FFS+	Traditional
PCO	Full	Capitation	Negotiated by case manager
PCP/Medical School	P/B/A	Capitation	Traditional
PCP/PCO	P/B/A	Capitation/SSO	Traditional
PCO	P/B/A	Capitation/SSO	Traditional
PCP	P/B/A	1. FFS 2. Capitation/SSO	Traditional
PHP	Full	Capitation	Negotiated by HMO/PHP
PCO	P/B/A	Capitation/SSO	Traditional
PCP/PCO	P/B/A	Capitation/SSO	Negotiated by HIO

Continued

Appendix 4.2 Continued

Program	*Date Established*	*Maximum Number Enrolled*	*Enrollment*	*Organizational Approach*
Utah's Choice of Health Care Delivery Plan	1982	25,000	Mandatory	State
Kitsap (WA) Sound Care Plan	1986	6,500	Mandatory	HIO
Washington Voluntary HMO Enrollment in Group Health Cooperative	1972	5,000	Voluntary	State
Wisconsin HMO Program	1984	111,000	Mandatory	State

Note:
PCP = Primary care physician
PCO = Primary care organization
PHP = Prepaid health plan
CM = Case manager
P/B/A = Primary care with specified brokering and authorizing duties
CAP = Capitated plan
FFS+ = Fee-for-service with case management fee
SSO = Shared savings opportunities

References

Buchanan, J., A. Leibowitz, J. Keesey, J. Mann, and C. Damberg. 1992. *Cost and Use of Capitated Medical Services: Evaluation of the Program for Prepaid Managed Health Care.* RAND/UCLA/Harvard Center for Health Care Financing Policy Research. Santa Monica, CA: RAND Corporation.

Freund, D. 1984. *Medicaid Reform: Four Studies of Case Management.* Washington, DC: American Enterprise Institute.

Freund, D., and R. Hurley. 1987. "Managed Care in Medicaid: Selected Issues in Program Origins, Design, and Research." *Annual Review of Public Health* 8: 137–63.

Hurley, R. 1986. "The Status of the Medicaid Competition Demonstrations." *Health Care Financing Review* 8(2): 65–75.

Hurley, R., and D. Freund. 1988. "A Typology of Medicaid Managed Care." *Medical Care* 26(8): 764–73.

National Governors' Association (NGA). 1985. *Prepaid and Managed Care Under Medicaid: Overview of Current Initiatives.* Washington, DC: The Association.

Case Manager Selection	*Service Range Responsibility*	*Case Manager Payment Method*	*Other Provider Payment*
PCP	P/B/A	FFS	Traditional
PCP/PCO	P/B/A	Capitation/SSO	Negotiated by HIO
PHP	Full	Capitation	Negotiated by case manager
PHP	Full	Capitation	Negotiated by case manager

Office of Research and Demonstration (ORD). 1987. *Medicaid Program Evaluation: Final Report.* Report No. MPE 9.2. Eds. J. Holahan, J. Bell, and G. S. Adler. Baltimore, MD: Health Care Financing Administration.

Research Triangle Institute (RTI). 1988. *Evaluation of the Medicaid Competition Demonstrations, Final Report.* Vol. 6, Administrative Costs. Contract No. HCFA-500-83-0050. Research Triangle Park, NC: Research Triangle Institute.

———. 1989. *Evaluation of the Medicaid Competition Demonstrations: Integrative Final Report.* Contract No. HCFA-500-83-0050. Research Triangle Park, NC: Research Triangle Institute.

SRI International. 1989. *Evaluation of the Arizona Health Care Cost Containment System: Final Report.* Contract No. HCFA-500-83-0027. Palo Alto, CA: SRI International.

Welch, W. P., A. Hillman, and M. Pauly. 1990. "Toward New Typologies for HMOs." *Milbank Memorial Fund Quarterly* 68(2): 221–43.

Chapter 5

Evaluating the Evidence: An Assessment of Methodologies

Public policy evaluation is a complex, expensive, and often contentious process. The experience of researchers in evaluating Medicaid PCCM programs sustains this tradition. From available documentation, we estimate that upwards of $15 million may have been expended to evaluate the 25 programs included in this study. There is, moreover, great diversity among the studies performed to date of Medicaid PCCM programs in terms of sponsorship, resources invested, data sources, level of analysis, and methodological rigor. Consequently, the validity and usefulness of the findings from these studies vary. More importantly, however, the studies represent an enormous volume of data that can be converted into usable knowledge only if it is adequately appraised and analyzed. Appraising the quality and usefulness of the various study findings is the focus of this chapter.

The chapter begins with a review of the principal sources of findings from all 25 evaluations, including some comments on the waiver application process.[1] We follow this overview with a discussion of a number of the key analytical challenges faced by those who evaluate Medicaid PCCM programs. Selection and interpretation problems relating to cost and utilization measures are then described and discussed. This discussion leads into a review of the methodological approaches employed in the 25 programs. We propose a set of criteria to assess methodological rigor in the studies. Finally, we present a general overview of the evidence, including the identification of a subset of programs that have a relatively higher level of validity and reliability. This methodologically stronger subset is given special attention in Chapter 7, in which we examine the findings from each individual program.

Data Sources and Sponsorship

As noted earlier, the 25 programs included in this study are a purposive sample from the universe of Medicaid PCCM initiatives. The programs were selected on the basis of having systematically collected evidence of program effects on the cost and use of services by Medicaid beneficiaries. We also imposed one additional condition for program selection into the study: the programs' own evaluation had to include, at a minimum, an evaluation of the impact on AFDC beneficiaries. This restriction was designed to ensure reasonable comparability of program enrollees across states. Moreover, AFDC eligibles are the largest group of Medicaid beneficiaries and the group most frequently enrolled in PCCM programs.

There are four major data sources for the impact analysis presented in this book; specific data sources for each site are described in the program summaries in the appendix. The data sources include the following:

1. Externally funded studies, typically sponsored by the federal government
2. External assessments funded by states to meet federal (HCFA) waiver requirements
3. State-produced assessments prepared internally for inclusion with waiver applications
4. Peer-reviewed articles appearing in the professional literature

Generally speaking, the externally funded studies were the best funded and most rigorous in design and implementation. Although there were some exceptions, those in the third category represented the least expensive and least methodologically rigorous studies.

Three major federally sponsored studies merit special comment: the MCD evaluation (RTI 1989), the MPE (ORD 1987), and the AHCCCS evaluation (SRI International 1989). The MCD evaluation included studies of several Section 1115 demonstration programs, of which seven are included in this analysis. The MPE, which examined early OBRA waiver experience, included six Section 1915b waiver programs, all of which are included in this study. Since the MPE incorporated information from existing studies (i.e., it did not do original data analysis), the source studies and later assessments from some of these programs have been separately included in our study. The AHCCCS evaluation studied the statewide experimental program implemented under a Section 1115 waiver that represented Arizona's initial entry into the Medicaid program. Two other major but smaller-scale studies also fall into the externally funded category: the Children's Medicaid Program of Suffolk County (New York) funded by the HCFA and the Hartford Foundation and the Wintringham and Bice (1985) study of Group Health Cooperative in Washington state funded by the National Center for Health Services Research (NCHSR) (subsequently the Agency for Health Care Policy and Research, AHCPR).

The second category of studies includes several state program evaluations, such as those in Pennsylvania, Washington State, Michigan, Ohio, and Colorado, that were incorporated into federal waiver and waiver renewal applications. Several of these studies incorporated sophisticated analytical designs.

The third category of studies includes internally prepared analyses that accompanied waiver documentation. Typically these studies have been far less extensive, and some have serious methodological limitations, although there are important exceptions to this norm, such as the studies conducted for Wisconsin and Kentucky.

The fourth category of information on the programs includes articles appearing in the professional literature. This source of information is often well documented regarding methodology and outcomes.

Because two categories of information comprise studies that were performed as part of the waiver application or waiver renewal process, it is important to comment on potentially confounding effects. A condition for waiver renewal for already operational programs is their ability to document ongoing cost-effectiveness. Therefore, study sponsors clearly had a vested interest in presenting findings that supported this assertion, since failure to do so could jeopardize the waiver request. This potential conflict of interest does not necessarily imply misrepresented or misleading analyses. It simply underscores that the methods adopted typically are designed to present program impact, especially relating to cost, in the most favorable light. There are many possible approaches to the estimation of cost savings, which make establishing cost-effectiveness as part of the waiver renewal application not especially difficult. Obviously, some approaches have greater validity than others. Some of the possible study weaknesses or threats to validity in the cost area include

- attributing apparent savings solely to the PCCM intervention without ruling out other contributing state or federal Medicaid program changes;
- arbitrarily selecting comparison or study groups, leading to the amplification of impact; and
- making questionable assumptions about expected levels of cost and use in the absence of the program intervention.

These and other issues are discussed later in more detail. However, there are important implications for the assessment of the individual study methodologies. There are also some significant policy implications regarding both the burdensomeness and the validity of the waiver renewal process.

The Evaluation Challenge

Evaluation of ongoing, real-time public programs presents many challenges to evaluators. Conducting an evaluation for programs as diverse and ambiguous as the Medicaid PCCM initiatives is even more problematic. Theoretical or conceptual models of case manager behavior have not been well developed, nor have expectations for gatekeepers customarily been well explicated. Program models have been viewed as idiosyncratic, and no unifying or organization classification systems have been widely accepted. Program managers have also offered differing explanations for what their programs have intended to do, such as containing costs, improving access, improving the coordination of care, or altering usual sites of care.

Coupled with this underdeveloped conceptualization of PCCM have been the difficulties associated with implementing theoretical designs within practical programs. Enormous time delays in implementing programs and acquiring data are well documented in the evaluation studies. These delays have caused many problems for program evaluators who are striving for timely and comparable results across sites that are at differing stages of implementation and readiness for evaluation. The programs have also experienced design slippage—the program implemented might differ markedly from the originally conceived design—thus necessitating changes in an already-ongoing evaluation. Finally, a lack of resources has hampered both program implementation and evaluation. The result often has been that the programs themselves have ended up suboptimized, and the rigor of resulting evaluations has been disappointing or compromised.

Evaluation design issues

Evaluation requires both science and art. In essence, the objective is to enable an analyst to study phenomenon systematically with the goal of understanding (i.e., explaining or predicting) both variation and the factors that might contribute to this variation. In another sense, evaluation can focus on the impact of a phenomenon on some events or occurrences, which, if the evaluation design is sufficiently robust, might enable the observer to infer a causal relationship. In our case, the question can be posed regarding the impact of PCCM on beneficiary cost and use experience, with the goal of establishing that it does or does not have an effect.

To accomplish this goal, evaluation designs for Medicaid PCCM must be developed that can both isolate the case management intervention and link it unambiguously to the observed outcomes while ruling out or at least controlling for other possible contributory factors. A few of the studies reported here lack even a rudimentary evaluation design, using only a simplistic analytical approach based on comparing postintervention program experience to unsubstantiated assertions of what the experience might have been if the program were absent. This design is implemented by simply drawing on prior levels of use or cost to project future trends.

A more customary method for addressing the research design task is to use a quasi-experimental approach (i.e., a contrast or comparison of similar groups that are differentially exposed to the phenomenon of interest) (Cook and Campbell 1979). For PCCM this comparison can be done before and after to explore the effect of "going into gatekeeping" (Hurley, Freund, and Taylor 1989). If a specified group (i.e., panel or cohort) of beneficiaries is carefully tracked during the transition from the unmanaged care preenrollment period to their enrollment with gatekeepers, a natural contrast is presented and, if no other changes occurred during this period, a case can be made that observed changes can be attributed to the intervention. The contrast can be further enhanced if the gatekeeper was the beneficiary's prior usual source of care and if it can be established that the health status of the beneficiary has not changed during the transition to gatekeeping. Both of these requirements can be addressed with statistical controls through multivariable models (Neter and Wasserman 1974).

An alternative methodology to accomplish a meaningful contrast is to select a comparison group of nonenrolled beneficiaries with similar characteristics whose use and cost experience can be compared with that of enrolled beneficiaries. Such a comparison can be cross-sectional or contemporaneous. In this case, differences observed can also be attributed with some confidence to the PCCM intervention. However, ensuring the similarities of the two groups via sampling or statistical methodologies is critical to the success of this design.

A still stronger design can be achieved if both before and after and comparison group approaches are included. This type of design controls for both (1) group or site differences and (2) historical or temporal changes that might otherwise contaminate findings. In this design, the rate of change in cost and use for enrollees is contrasted with the rate of change for nonenrollees, and this difference is identified as the program effect. Sampling techniques and statistical controls can further strengthen the robustness of such findings.

Theoretically, of course, the ideal evaluation design would include the use of random assignment of beneficiaries to primary care gatekeepers. This approach would remove the threat of bias due to nonrandom selection of either the gatekeeper opportunity or the specific selection of a gatekeeper. Pure experiments, however, are extremely rare for public programs in general and for Medicaid PCCM programs in particular. This situation is due in part to the desire of program managers at a minimum to allow beneficiaries the opportunity to select the PCP who will manage their care. There would also be the disadvantage of random assignment potentially disrupting existing patient-provider relationships. One of the programs included in this study (Minnesota—Hennepin County) employed random assignment as part of the research design to determine who would be in a gatekeeper program but allowed beneficiaries to choose their own gatekeeper. The selection bias issue is particularly important in voluntary programs because beneficiaries who participate in the program might be systematically different from those who choose to remain in the regular, unmanaged Medicaid program. A recent study that employed random assignment to examine selection bias in voluntary HMO enrollment programs in Medicaid has been performed by the RAND Corporation (Buchanan et al. 1992). In that study an experimental design was employed to create four study groups: (1) random assignment to FFS, (2) random assignment to HMO coverage, (3) self-selection into FFS, and (4) self-selection into an HMO. Although detailed findings from the RAND study were not available for inclusion among the 25 programs presented in this study, preliminary results are included in the impact discussion in Chapter 7.

The preceding discussion focuses on the internal validity or reliability of the evaluation findings (Campbell and Stanley 1963). An equally compelling research design concern for both researchers and policymakers is the external validity or generalizability of the findings (Cook and Campbell 1979). At a minimum, evaluation findings should be drawn from a representative group of beneficiaries so that the evaluation is able to assess the total program. This generalizability aspect is problematic when evaluation designs are adopted for subgroups that do not fully reflect the total covered population. For example, among the studies examined, a number of the before and after analyses looked only at persons continuously eligible for Medicaid for two full years. Such an approach fails to appraise how gatekeeping programs might affect persons who are newly eligible or eligible for only part of the study period. Though reliability might be high in these studies, they are lacking in programwide generalizability.

A variable that can strongly affect both internal and external validity of evaluation results is program maturation. The ages of the programs reviewed in this study vary substantially, as do the points in time when evaluation evidence was collected and analyzed. This fact means that in some cases mature, stable programs are being evaluated while in other cases program effects are being evaluated after perhaps only a year of operation, with the programs still on a definite learning curve. Almost no studies have rigorous longitudinal designs that permit a valid assessment of learning-curve effects. Thus, reliability for the studies conducted early in the program's history might be questioned, because detected effects might subsequently either evaporate or intensify. Likewise, comparing well-established programs to programs early in their implementation is also potentially misleading. Some of the implications of this problem are discussed in subsequent chapters.

Evaluation data issues

Regardless of the elegance of the evaluation design adopted, its utility in isolating and demonstrating program effects depends on the acquisition of data that have both relevance and integrity. Evaluators must specify the data they need by identifying the hypothesized effects for PCCM. The hypotheses, in turn, originate in the conceptual or behavioral model that underlies the intervention. Most programs have used a general model that includes expectations that gatekeeper programs will reduce or control costs and restrict (though not impede) access. As already noted, however, this general model has not been adequately elaborated to the point where it can anticipate the actual dynamics of gatekeeping. For example, some of the subtle and not-so-subtle distinctions among gatekeeper programs, such as the use of risk-sharing, have not been used to develop more refined hypotheses. Furthermore, the level of detail in readily available data generally is not adequate to support investigation at these levels of distinction.

The need to identify relevant and sufficiently detailed data sources has led evaluators toward two principal data sources: (1) primary data collection via consumer surveys and (2) secondary data analysis, typically from administrative or claims data. Each source has certain associated strengths and weaknesses in terms of ease of collection, intrusiveness, level of detail, interpretability, etc. Both sources are susceptible to measurement error and to response and reporting bias. Both sources also necessitate careful construction of measures of utilization and costs that are meaningful and responsive to the hypothesized effects of PCCM, as differentially defined by various program managers. Several program evaluations have used both primary and secondary data to attempt to triangulate particular program effects, such as reduction in unnecessary emergency department use.

Since the focus of this study is on cost and use experience under Medicaid PCCM, secondary or claims-based data are the source of much of the available evidence. This means, however, that our analyses rely on data submitted for purposes other than program evaluation. Specifically, Medicaid claims are processed for payment and manifest the accompanying strengths and weaknesses of a bill-paying data-processing system. Wide variation exists in how the evaluators have chosen to use these data. For the purpose of supporting before and after or comparison group contrasts, some evaluators have chosen to assess effects for cost and use by summarizing expenditures in various service categories. Other evaluators have used enumeration at the procedure level to accumulate volume of services and through this approach have developed use measures of procedures per beneficiary, by selected service categories. Both of these approaches are appealingly simple, since Medicaid agencies have federal reporting requirements that specify the accumulation of data in this fashion. These approaches represent efforts of states to minimize the reporting burden, as well as the burden of developing documentation to support waiver-renewal applications.

More sophisticated person-level data bases have been developed in several studies, frequently through external financial support. These data bases convert claims data into intuitively meaningful measures of visits or encounters, such as physician office visits or emergency department visits, that permit more refined estimates of the dynamics of gatekeeping that include the place of service or the specialty of the provider. Person-level data can also permit the separation of volume-of-service changes from cost per unit of services or total expenditures. These data can identify whether delivery system patterns in gatekeeping are discernibly different from those in regular Medicaid. For example, the MCDs adopted a two-part model developed by RAND for the health insurance experiment (Duan et al. 1983 and 1984) to assess whether gatekeeping differentially affects the probability of use and use-for-users in certain services categories. Interesting effects with regard to emergency department gatekeeping have been reported using this model on the MCD data (Hurley, Freund, and Taylor 1989).

Perhaps the single most difficult and controversial of data issues in Medicaid PCCM programs has been the lack of reliable data from programs that pay either gatekeepers or HMOs/PHPs through capitation. The use of this payment method removes the incentive from providers to submit encounter- or service-level data conscientiously. In the extreme case of staff model HMOs, there might be no claims or bills for services since the physicians and health care providers are paid a salary. However, some type of service or encounter reporting system might be in place. For PCPs now covered by capitation for primary care services, one of the incentives offered to them might even have been liberation from detailed billing. The price paid by the state in granting this freedom to providers is the loss of the transparency of service delivery patterns as found under FFS-paid care. In fact, however, there seems to be little, if any, decrease in paperwork or reporting systems faced by providers or the states under these arrangements.

PCCM program developers have defined and addressed this problem differently. In some cases the lack of encounter- or service-level detail is accepted as a consequence of payment methods. Program officials might impose some alternative aggregate reporting requirements on participating providers or plans. In other cases, providers might be required to submit claims-like service-level encounter forms, commonly referred to as pseudo- or dummy claims, to track utilization. However, it might be inappropriate to place more than relatively low confidence in these types of claims given the expectation of substantial underreporting. Finally, several of the large demonstration programs were required to specify that providers submit pseudoclaims as a condition of participation in the program. These pseudoclaims were then to be processed and used to examine program effects. Despite this requirement, however, experience with this requirement has been uneven and generally disappointing, with several programs failing to generate adequate encounter data for the first several years of the program.

There have been a few attempts in the larger evaluations to assess the extent of underreporting in pseudoclaims, but no studies have adjusted for its impact. The MCD evaluation used several relational analyses (e.g., the ratio of physician visits covered under capitation to FFS-paid drug prescriptions) to assess underreporting. Validation studies of underreporting have also been conducted in the AHCCCS study (SRI International 1989). To date, the most exhaustive study of underreporting was conducted for the Suffolk County, New York, evaluation, in which reported encounters were matched with medical record documentation (Hohlen et al. 1990). This approach represents a costly but highly reliable methodology. This analysis found underreporting to be in the range of 10 to 15 percent. However, like many of the other features of this carefully planned and implemented demonstration, it is doubtful that findings can be easily generalized to other program evaluations.

Approaches to data analysis

The analytical approaches adopted in the program evaluations are of necessity closely linked to the evaluation designs selected and data sources available. Customarily, there is a compensating effect between the resources required to develop an elegant research design and the required resources for and sophistication of the statistical analysis. Straightforward analyses are possible in carefully crafted designs, while complex statistical adjustments and controls might be called for when a design is weak or nonexistent. An example of the former would be the MCD evaluations of Santa Barbara or Monterey counties, California, while the use of the complex grade of membership (GOM) methodology for the HealthPASS program typifies the latter (Woodbury and Manton 1982). However, several of the evaluations have neither characteristic, employing only minimal designs with limited analytical approaches.

As mentioned above, the level of detail of data and its presentation vary across the program evaluations included in this study. A number of programs sum aggregate use or cost experience for samples and then divide these by the number of eligibles or eligible-months in the sample. This approach can be done for all eligibles or, in several programs, separately for subgroups of eligibles such as AFDC adults and AFDC children. These are, in effect, mean levels of use for entire populations. Because they do not adjust for variation in the duration of eligibility for individual persons, they are subject to biases due to nonnormal distributions. They also do not permit multivariate analyses in which individual levels of beneficiary attributes are controlled or adjusted for before testing for case management effects. This situation can be particularly problematic when comparison groups come from sites that have some substantial differences in factors affecting the use of medical care. An example would be programs that have been implemented in primarily urban areas and are not matched to any other equally urbanized comparison groups. In some cases age and gender stratification has been used to create more homogeneous classes for contrast purposes. In particular, cost data for several programs have been derived at this more aggregated level. This issue is discussed in detail later in this chapter.

Conducting an analysis with person-level data in terms of demographic and utilization statistics overcomes a number of limitations, although difficulties in constructing appropriate analysis files are correspondingly greater. Although data on personal characteristics contained in claims and eligibility files are limited, they can include such key measures as duration of eligibility or enrollment, age, gender, race, and the extent of other (non-Medicaid) insurance coverage. All of these characteristics can have a bearing on levels of use and cost.

Although to date infrequently used, these data files can also provide important detailed information on the procedural content of visits with and without gatekeeping and the proportion of an enrollee's care that is directly rendered by gatekeepers versus other providers. More exacting and reliable estimates of the presence or absence of selection bias in these programs can be conducted if person-level data are available, although the absence of true measures of health status in claims data remains problematic. Prior health care utilization (when preenrollment data are available) is the surrogate commonly adopted for health status.

With respect to statistical testing, a number of the evaluations omit tests of significance to evaluate the meaningfulness of findings. In some cases the tests could not be done given the analytical approach. In other cases they might have been viewed as unnecessary, with evaluators focusing on the substantive implications of differences rather than on their statistical significance. Despite the apparent deficiencies implied by the omission of significance testing, it must be noted that the findings from these studies were deemed sufficiently documented by federal waiver renewal authorities. More generally, they can be viewed as part of the uneven but cumulative evidence that has been produced across the 25 programs in this study.

Bivariate contrasts from before and after or demonstration/comparison groups have been commonly employed, as have multivariate models of use that control for various person-level characteristics while testing for intervention effects. In the latter models, ordinary least squares (OLS) regressions have been used to estimate mean levels of use, and limited dependent variable regressions (e.g., logit and probit) have been used to estimate probabilities of use and the factors influencing them. A few programs have employed simple trend analysis, which may include changes dubiously attributed to the primary care intervention. Changes in this case would be any observed differences between expected and actual use and cost experience. (A notable exception to this was the analysis for the Kentucky program, which used an interrupted time series approach with procedure-level, rather than person-level, data.) Finally, several programs susceptible to selection bias, either into a voluntary program or among plans in a mandatory program, have analyzed this effect using sophisticated econometric modeling techniques (see, for example, Volume 8 of the MCD evaluation [RTI 1988]).

Selecting Outcome Measures of Use and Cost

Many features and facets of PCCM have been studied among the 25 programs incorporated into this study. In addition to effects on cost and use, other areas include beneficiary satisfaction, service accessibility, quality of care, provider participation, and provider satisfaction, as well as the host of contextual factors that have been examined through elaborate case studies. However, the focus of this integrative study has been limited to cost and use for several reasons. First, although almost all studies report at least on these two outcomes, relatively few report on the full spectrum outlined above. In addition, data on these effects must be reported for virtually all programs in their waiver applications. Given the goals of these programs, answers to the questions of impact on cost and use are fundamental to the evaluation of the desirability of continued expansion of the PCCM strategy. We also hypothesize that differences in program designs or prototypes will be detected for the areas of cost and use effects, whereas differences might not be detectable for other effects. Finally, a higher degree of objective comparison among programs is possible with cost and use measures than would be possible in areas that are more difficult to measure, such as beneficiary satisfaction, quality of care, or provider participation and satisfaction.

Measuring utilization effects

Although many features of PCCM effects on use are of potential interest, the selection of which features to examine is limited by the availability of data. The hypothesized effects of gatekeeping on ambulatory and inpatient use were introduced in Chapter 2. Four types of ambulatory use are examined in this section: physician services; emergency department services; ancillary service use, primarily referring to laboratory and x-ray services; and prescription drugs. Effects on inpatient use are examined through numbers of admissions or days of care.

Physician services are measured as counts of visits for the entire sample (the use rate); the proportion of the sample with at least one physician visit (the probability of use); and the number of visits for users (use-for-users). A few programs also provided counts of the number of procedures rendered by physicians as a measure of physician services, or summed the expenditures made to individual physicians and reported this amount as a proxy for physician service use.

Each of the measures provides somewhat different information, but each also permits an assessment of how the provision of physician services might have changed due to the gatekeeper intervention. Other measures, such as the place of service, the specialty of physicians, and authorized versus unauthorized referrals are available for a few programs. Such measures allow for richer views of the dynamics of gatekeeping but have limited availability across programs, making comparisons and generalizations difficult.

The same types of measures generally are available for other ambulatory services, although only about half of the programs reported any evidence regarding ancillary and prescription use. The methods of measurement for both of these indicators varied, especially in the case of ancillary use. Some studies counted laboratory or x-ray procedures by way of procedural codes, while others only counted visits for which there were indications that laboratory or x-ray services were provided. In both cases, a high correlation between ancillary and physician service use was noted in a number of the studies, as discussed in the next chapter. Prescription use has typically been represented by a count of prescriptions per beneficiary. A limitation of this method is that it does not reflect counts of units dispensed nor the cost of the drugs prescribed. A few programs report prescription drug expenditures which, to a certain extent, provide a more aggregated picture of changes in drug-prescribing experience.

The measures of emergency department use are generally widely available and highly informative regarding gatekeeper effects under

PCCM. Several programs, however, were unable to separate emergency department use from other types of hospital outpatient use. Changes in overall outpatient visits cannot be solely attributed to emergency department reductions since a number of gatekeeper programs achieve a high level of site shifting (i.e., moving care from outpatient clinics to physician offices or to health clinics). It should also be noted that care provided in health clinics and, to a lesser extent, PHPs, often lacked the detailed coding necessary to identify fully the details of the encounter.

The extreme illustration of differential reporting is in the underreporting problem noted earlier, where some providers or plans submit no reports at the service level. For capitated plans or organizations, the most reliable reported information might be services provided by external contractors such as hospitals and emergency departments with whom the plans or organizations engage through discrete transactions. For this reason, inpatient use is probably the most reliably reported measure across all the programs. Inpatient care commonly is examined in terms of enumerating admissions and tabulating days of care. However, it is also apparent that some programs have reached questionable conclusions by claiming that observed reductions in inpatient use are solely attributable to the PCCM strategy. This point is discussed further in the next chapter.

Measuring cost effects

Measuring cost effects might be more aptly described as measuring cost savings since, at least for the waiver applications, the issue and analyses typically have been framed in this manner.[2] In some instances only savings have been reported, not savings as a percentage of expenditures, which underscores the advocacy logic that has gone into many analyses. Despite this concern, there are some important assumptions and difficult problems to be addressed in devising evaluations of the impact of gatekeeper interventions on program costs and expenditures. These problems include, (1) Whose perspective is being adopted to estimate savings? (2) What will be the point of reference with which actual expenditures will be contrasted? and (3) How do these actual expenditures compare to what might have been expended? These problems, moreover, are also confounded by program design issues.

One way to examine how assumptions play a role in estimating cost effects is to consider the measures of costs that could be used to highlight interesting contrasts, as shown in Exhibit 5.1.

With regard to the program prototypes, the following comparisons are appropriate for assessing cost effects.

For studies evaluating Type 1 programs, the contrasts of interests would be A (plus the case management fee, if appropriate) versus D or E depending on whether a before and after (D) or comparison group design

Exhibit 5.1 Possible Cost Measures

Intervention Group Expenditures

A. FFS expenditures made for beneficiaries in gatekeeper programs
B. Capitation payments (plus FFS expenditures, if any) for beneficiaries in gatekeeper programs
C. FFS equivalent costs for beneficiaries in gatekeeper programs whose care was paid by capitation

Comparison Group Expenditures

D. Estimated or expected expenditures for beneficiaries in gatekeeper programs if they had not been enrolled
E. FFS expenditures made for beneficiaries in comparison groups

(E) is employed. Evaluations using both design features would use information from both D and E.

Type 2 and 3 program evaluations have similar contrasts available, though B rather than A would be used to assess actual expenditures in the intervention program.

All PCCM programs potentially include another contrast of interest—C versus D or E. This contrast provides a picture of how the gatekeeper program actually affected service delivery use as measured by the (imputed) resources consumed by beneficiaries. It answers more directly the question whether service delivery was different under the gatekeeper program from what would have been observed in its absence, or what was observed in a comparison group. Finally, the contrast of C versus B assesses the adequacy of the capitation rates paid to gatekeepers as compared to the Medicaid-priced package of services provided. The difference could arguably be viewed, from the HMO's perspective, as the extent to which it was overpaid or underpaid (and vice versa from the state's perspective).

Most evaluations included in our study estimate cost effects based on the use of either A or B as contrasted with D or E. Several of them report these data aggregated to the entire enrolled population rather than on an individual person-level basis. The adoption of this approach, as noted above, leads to contrasts among heterogeneous groups such as urban versus rural populations. In other cases in which trend lines are extended from preimplementation periods several years into the future, the implicit assumption is that no other changes have occurred, either in the study population or in Medicaid program eligibility or policies as a whole. This is, to say the least, a heroic assumption that casts doubt on the reliability of the estimates made for these programs.

Another overarching problem in estimating and presenting cost savings is the issue of whose perspective is to be adopted. Most typically, the vantage point is that of the state Medicaid agency, although several programs also enumerate the extent of savings that is represented in the federal matching percentage.

Whose perspective is adopted takes on added importance when the state agency is contracting with either HIOs or directly with HMOs or PHPs (Type 3 programs). In these cases, the state is paying to the HIO, or the HMO or PHP, a capitation payment that is computed on the basis of an estimate of expected FFS expenditures that would have been made had the capitated gatekeeper program not been implemented, as in D above. This rate is then discounted (perhaps after a stop-loss fund deduction is made) from 2.5 percent up to 10 percent to ensure that the program expenditures net of administrative costs will not exceed what would have been spent in an FFS environment. For the purpose of demonstrating cost-effectiveness in waiver applications, states then claim the net discount as their savings.

In fact, most programs do not have sufficiently detailed data to go much beyond this basis for estimating savings, in part because of the lack of encounter data. Consequently, virtually all states either using the HIO option or directly administering Type 3 HMO or PHP programs report cost savings. Although these savings are true savings in every respect, they are not directly comparable to savings computed from Type 1 or Type 2 programs, in which the savings reflect actual reductions in services consumed or changes in provider behavior. In effect, the savings associated with contracting with HMOs or PHPs might or might not result from differences in the volume of services rendered. They could be due simply to the willingness of these types of organizations to provide equivalent care for what turns out to be a lower price. No evaluation to date of Medicaid PCCM programs has attempted to answer this question directly.

Capitated Type 3 programs also present another subtle and significant cost analysis problem. Because newly eligible Medicaid beneficiaries cannot be instantaneously enrolled in HMOs or PHPs, it is not unusual for them to incur some medical expenses that are paid for by FFS Medicaid during the preenrollment window. When use or cost experience is subsequently analyzed for the period of enrollment, this preenrollment experience might not be properly attributed to the individual beneficiary. Because many newly eligible persons might use a substantial number of services during preenrollment, total use calculated only for the period of enrollment will be significantly understated. Moreover, the capitation rates paid to plans might be excessive if they are not adjusted for preenrollment use. A vivid example of this effect was observed in the AHCCCS evaluation, where for the initial years of this Type 3 program, nearly 20 percent of service expenditures was for FFS care (SRI International 1989, p. 19). Only person-level analyses can adequately control for this type of program leakage.

Summarizing Program Evaluation Features

Detailed evaluation features for the 25 programs are presented in the appendix. The selection of data sources was based on using the best available evaluation information. This approach means that where both waiver and other sources were available, we selected the more rigorously performed studies if they contained cost and use findings. For example, in the case of the MCD evaluations, the sources selected were the site-specific evaluations rather than state waiver applications. We discuss these features briefly and describe the range of variation on each in the sections that follow.

Program years evaluated

Of the 25 programs, 20 were still operational in 1991 with the oldest programs having seven to eight years of experience. Given claims processing lags and waiver renewal cycles, no program had more than six years of operational experience available for analysis. A high proportion of programs had detailed evaluation data only from the first full year of operation. Programs in five states had up to five to six years of experience, but none had strong longitudinal studies. Two states had more rigorous studies that offer some insight into the sustainability of program effects.

Data sources

A total of 19 programs used claims or pseudoclaims to develop measures of cost and use as described earlier. Data sources for the remaining 6 sites included, in most cases, consumer surveys or other aggregate reports from intermediaries or PHPs. Several programs used combinations of data sources. Evaluations in 3 sites attempted to assess systematically the extent of underreporting in encounter data for Type 2 and Type 3 programs. However, several other evaluations acknowledged the likely presence of underreporting and thus the unreliability of estimates conditioned on their use. Other evaluations used only summary data provided by PHPs because of a lack of confidence in the existing encounter data.

Representativeness of the study group

The representativeness of the study group is critical to generalizing the findings to the entire Medicaid-eligible population. For approximately half of the mandatory programs, representativeness was met through a random sampling strategy. Representativeness was problematic in a few of these programs because before and after design studies were performed only with data for continuously eligible beneficiaries. The representativeness of voluntary programs could not be assessed for the eligible population as a whole without an analysis of selection bias, which is discussed below.

Comparison groups

Out of the 25 programs, 20 provided a comparison group of nonenrollees or a preenrollment panel. One analysis actually used two comparison groups, an in-county and an out-of-county group. The key question regarding comparison groups is, in fact, their comparability. This basic issue posed problems in states that targeted gatekeeping to urban areas and thus were left with only nonurban areas from which to create comparison groups. Other sites employed actual beneficiary experience statewide or synthetically created comparison groups. Because the mandatory program in Arizona was statewide, it was necessary to use a comparison group of beneficiaries in New Mexico for some of the analyses. Generally, however, using out-of-state comparison groups is particularly undesirable due to state-by-state variation in Medicaid eligibility requirements and covered services.

Before and after contrasts

Fifteen programs reported using before and after analyses. Another two used trend analyses that incorporated preimplementation data into the estimates of cost and use effects. Approximately 12 programs used combined before and after and comparison group designs. In several cases, the before and after and the comparison group contrasts were refined further via statistical techniques.

Person-level data

The use experience of individual beneficiaries was the unit of analysis in 17 of the 25 programs, with the remainder presenting only aggregated use, which was divided by eligible persons, or person-months divided by years of eligibility, to arrive at rates of use. Relatively few programs used person-level data to compute cost savings; most relied on aggregate accumulations or estimates of expenditures.

Statistical adjustments

Fourteen programs used person-level files and characteristics to adjust or control the analyses. In effect, the evaluators used these adjustments with, or as a substitute for, various before and after or comparison group designs to equate the contrasted groups on available attributes. The most commonly used variables were age and gender. Only about half of the programs presented separate estimates of effects on AFDC adults and AFDC children.

Statistical tests for differences

Formal tests for statistically significant differences between an intervention group's experience and a contrast group's experience were found in 14 of the 25 studies. Depending on the analyses, *t*-tests, *F*-tests, X^2, or *p*-values were used.

Selection bias tests and adjustments

Studies for four voluntary programs examined evidence of selection bias with regard to enrollment. The evaluation of one mandatory program examined selection bias with regard to plan selection. There was only one voluntary program that did not have data on selection bias. As noted earlier, none of the estimates of program effects attempted to adjust for any identified selection bias.

Cost savings calculations and contrasts

Wide variation in methods is observed for this measure, as described in the program summaries. Among the most basic, least rigorous approaches was to establish historical FFS expenditures from a designated period before implementation, project a trend, compare this trend line to actual expenditures, and attribute lower-than-expected expenditures to program savings. The most common technique in Type 1 and Type 2 program prototypes was to compare rates of changes observed in intervention groups to nonenrolled comparison groups and suggest that the intervention was the sole source of the reductions. The rigor of the designs and analyses in terms of controlling for other potential contributing factors added varying degrees persuasiveness to these assertions. As previously described, the Type 3 programs typically computed cost savings by describing the setting of capitation rates discounted from expected FFS expenditures and then multiplying this discount times the number of enrollees.

Summary

The range of variation in the methods, validity, and reliability of the findings from the 25 programs makes summarization difficult. The program summaries in the appendix provide details on the individual features of each program evaluation.

As an alternative, we propose a subset of 12 programs to represent those programs for which the most robust evaluations exist. Overall, these programs appear to merit confidence in the methodologies employed to assess program cost and use impacts. This confidence does not necessarily ensure that the findings are the most informative, however, given variations in program size, maturity, and the availability of data of interest; we only suggest that they represent a relatively higher degree of methodological rigor. The PCCM programs included in this category are shown in Exhibit 5.2.

Each of the selected studies offered, at a minimum, a detailed before and after or comparison group analysis. Each conducted person-level analyses, with the exception of two studies, which compensated by using either age and gender stratification or a combination of analytical approaches. All 12 programs presented both cost and use results. Thus, while every one of the studies contained acknowledged and perhaps significant limitations, they represent the most reliable sources of analytical findings regarding PCCM.

The requirement for both cost and use data for inclusion among the 12 ''better'' studies listed in Exhibit 5.2 meant the omission of otherwise well-done studies such as the Minnesota—Hennepin County Program study (which has no cost data) and the Arizona AHCCCS program evaluation (which has unreliable use data).

The identification of these methodologically stronger programs is useful in the next chapter for focusing the discussion of the evidence on cost and use impacts, which is presented first for all 25 programs and subse-

Exhibit 5.2 Selected Programs with More Methodologically Rigorous Studies

Monterey County (CA) Health Initiative
Santa Barbara County (CA) Health Initiative
Kentucky Patient Access and Care System
Louisville (KY) Citicare Program
Missouri Physician Sponsors Plan
Missouri Prepaid Health Plan Program
New Jersey Medicaid Personal Physician Plan
Erie County (NY) Physician Case Management Program (Children)
Children's Medicaid Program of Suffolk County (NY)
Dayton (OH) Area Health Plan
Utah's Choice of Health Care Delivery Programs
Washington Voluntary HMO Enrollment in Group Health Cooperative

quently from the subset of 12 programs. As the findings are discussed, results from the subset merit greater attention and weight for drawing conclusions about the effects of PCCM in Medicaid. Results from the other programs, however, are also informative. The similarities and disparities noted in them, as compared with the more rigorously evaluated programs, provide further evidence to corroborate or contrast in building a usable body of knowledge on PCCM.

Notes

1. The detailed program summaries in the appendix beginning on page 127 provide specific data sources for each program referenced in this chapter.
2. In actuality, the analyses focus on changes in *expenditures,* not on changes in actual *resource costs,* which are virtually impossible to ascertain in the health sector.

References

Buchanan, J., A. Leibowitz, J. Keesey, J. Mann, and C. Damberg. 1992. *Cost and Use of Capitated Medical Services: Evaluation of the Program for Prepaid Managed Health Care.* RAND/UCLA/Harvard Center for Health Care Financing Policy Research. Santa Monica, CA: RAND Corporation.

Campbell, D., and J. Stanley. 1963. *Experimental and Quasi-Experimental Design for Research.* Chicago: Rand McNally.

Cook, T. D., and D. T. Campbell. 1979. *Quasi-Experimentation: Design and Analysis Issues for Field Settings.* Boston: Houghton-Mifflin.

Duan, N., W. Manning, N. Morris, and J. Newhouse. 1983. "A Comparison of Alternative Models for the Demand for Medical Care." *Journal of Business and Economic Statistics* 1(2): 115–26.

———. 1984. "Choosing Between the Sample-Selection Model and the Multi-Part Mode." *Journal of Business and Economic Statistics* 2(1): 283–89.

Hohlen, M., L. Manheim, G. Fleming, S. Davidson, B. Yudkowsky, S. Wermer, and G. Wheatley. 1990. "Access to Office-Based Physicians Under Capitation Reimbursement and Medicaid Case Management: Findings from the Children's Medicaid Program." *Medical Care* 28(1): 59–68.

Hurley, R., D. Freund, and D. Taylor. 1989. "Emergency Room Use and Primary Care Case Management: Evidence from Four Medicaid Demonstration Programs." *American Journal of Public Health* 79(7): 843–46.

Neter, J., and W. Wasserman. 1974. *Applied Linear Statistical Models: Regression, Analysis of Variance, and Experimental Designs.* Homewood, IL: Richard D. Irwin, Inc.

Office of Research and Demonstrations (ORD). 1987. *Medicaid Program Evaluation: Final Report.* Report No. MPE 9.2. Eds. J. Holahan, J. Bell, and G. S. Adler. Baltimore, MD: Health Care Financing Administration.

Research Triangle Institute (RTI). 1988. Evaluation of the Medicaid Competition Demonstrations, Final Report. Vol. 8, *Enrollment Choice and Biased Selection*. Contract No. HCFA-500-83-0050. Research Triangle Park, NC: Research Triangle Institute.

———. 1989. *Evaluation of the Medicaid Competition Demonstrations: Integrative Final Report*. Contract No. HCFA-500-83-0050. Research Triangle Park, NC: Research Triangle Institute.

SRI International. 1989. *Evaluation of the Arizona Health Care Cost Containment System: Final Report*. Contract No. HCFA-500-83-0027. Palo Alto, CA: SRI International.

Wintringham, K., and T. Bice. 1985. "Effects of Turnover on Use of Services by Medicaid Beneficiaries in a Health Maintenance Organization." *The Group Health Journal* 6(1): 12–18.

Woodbury, M. A., and K. G. Manton. 1982. "A New Procedure for Analysis of Medical Classification." *Methods of Information in Medicine* 21: 210–20.

Chapter 6

Reviewing the Evidence for Effects on Cost and Use

Wide disparities in program designs and evaluation methodologies employed in the 25 programs included in this study were described in the preceding two chapters. This chapter addresses differences and similarities in program findings and outcomes relating to the cost and use of health services. The chapter begins with a review of the hypotheses regarding PCCM and gatekeeping proposed in Chapter 2. The hypotheses are examined in this chapter in the context of the programs. We present findings both for all programs and for those suggested to have the most reliable and valid data. We also examine the findings by four of the key features in the typology. Finally, we summarize evidence for each of the three program prototypes. The focus is both on the broad patterns of effects and on the range of variation noted in these effects. A discussion of the evidence is presented in Chapter 7.

Hypothesized Outcomes

The PCCM model developed in Chapter 2 attempted to present a comprehensive picture of the effects of primary care gatekeeping. However, given the modest amount of data available from the programs included in this study and the focus on cost and use effects only, the scope of the hypotheses proposed for testing was limited. The hypotheses are restated as follows:

Hypothesis 1: The effect of primary care gatekeeping on utilization will be mixed, and will depend on the payment mechanism.

Hypothesis 1a: Under FFS the effect of primary care gatekeeping will be to increase the total number of physician visits.

Hypothesis 1b: If physicians are paid on an at-risk basis, the effect will be to decrease the total number of physician visits.

Hypothesis 2: Emergency department use will be lower under all gatekeeper program designs because of a guaranteed relationship with a PCP and because emergency department visits for other than true emergencies will not be reimbursed unless formally authorized by the gatekeeper.

Hypothesis 3: Ancillary and prescription use will be lower in gatekeeper programs.

Hypothesis 3a: In PCCM programs that place gatekeepers at financial risk, ancillary and prescription use will be even lower.

Hypothesis 4: Inpatient use will be unchanged or slightly lower in primary gatekeeper programs due to better care coordination.

Hypothesis 4a: PCCM programs with financially at-risk gatekeepers and PHPs are more likely to reduce inpatient use.

Hypothesis 5: Primary care gatekeeper programs will result in small but significant reductions in overall program expenditures.

Hypothesis 5a: Expenditures may be larger in PCCM programs that employ financial risk-sharing with the gatekeepers.

We do not include several critical hypotheses regarding the effects of PCCM on utilization because of limited data availability. These hypotheses include information on beneficiaries' prior access to and affiliation with PCPs; evidence of an impact on specialist referrals or the substitution of primary care for specialists; the concentration of care with gatekeepers; and longitudinal effects on the utilization of health care. All these areas have received some prior attention in the literature and, as discussed in Chapter 8, clearly merit further exploration.

Summary of Findings

The findings of program effects for each of the five use measures and the single measure of costs are summarized in Table 6.1. Each measure is discussed in the following sections.

Table 6.1 Summary of Program Effects: Overall Results from 25 Programs

	Increase	*Decrease*	*Mixed/ No Change*	*Unknown*
Physician visits	11 (44%)	8 (32%)	5 (20%)	1 (4%)
Emergency department use	1 (4%)	13 (52%)	2 (8%)	9 (36%)
Ancillary services	2 (8%)	7 (28%)	3 (12%)	13 (52%)
Prescription drug use	3 (12%)	11 (44%)	2 (8%)	9 (36%)
Inpatient use	1 (4%)	17 (68%)	5 (20%)	2 (8%)
Costs	2 (8%)	19 (76%)	3 (12%)	1 (4%)

Note: Numbers indicate the number of programs; percentages are a percent of all programs in that category. Percentages might not add up to 100 due to rounding.

Physician visits

As proposed in Hypothesis 1, findings are mixed for this measure, although the large number of programs reporting increases in physician visits is notable. Increases in physician visits range from 6 to 37 percent, with four other programs reporting increases in the 20 to 30 percent range. These increases suggest that access to physician services in these sites has not been impeded and might in fact be enhanced. Decreases reported in physician use ranged from very slight decreases to nearly 20 percent for two programs, although underreporting of physician visits was likely for these two programs. Two other programs that have been reported in detail (the Missouri PSP program and the New Jersey program—see Freund et al. 1989), suggest that reductions in physician visits are the net result of reductions in specialist visits and increases in primary care visits. The sites without substantial changes also may have experienced such competing effects.

Emergency department visits

The findings regarding Hypothesis 2, testing the effect of primary care gatekeeping on emergency department visits, are highly consistent with expectations and prior published results. The magnitude of reductions is substantial, as shown by individual program in Table 6.2.

The full evidence of reductions, however, is probably even stronger than reflected in this list of programs. Several of the programs listed with "unknown" emergency department effects reported sharp reductions in outpatient visits but did not separate emergency department visits from other hospital outpatient visits. Since outpatient visits might also be lower

Table 6.2 Reductions in Emergency Department Use for 11 Programs

Programs Showing Reductions in Emergency Department Use	*Percentage Reduction in Emergency Department Use*
Missouri Physician Sponsors Plan	35 (children) 50 (adult)
Missouri Prepaid Health Plan Program	35 (children) 44 (adult)
New Jersey Medicaid Personal Physician Plan	37 (children) 43 (adult)
Louisville (KY) Citicare Program	40
Monterey County (CA) Health Initiative	35
Dayton (OH) Area Health Plan	30
Santa Barbara County (CA) Health Initiative	28 (children) 30 (adult)
Wisconsin HMO Program	25
Erie County (NY) Physician Case Management Program (Children)	22
Michigan Medicaid Physician Sponsor Plan	20
Utah's Choice of Health Care Delivery Programs	11

due to the shifting of primary care to physician offices, it is not possible to attribute reductions to a reduction in emergency department visits alone. The two programs that reported emergency department use as unchanged appear to have already had emergency department use well in check with most program beneficiaries already affiliated with a PCP before program implementation. Only one increase in emergency department use was reported, and no supporting evidence indicated a reason for this anomalous finding.

Ancillary services and prescription use

The findings with respect to these two types of use are reported less frequently than are physician and emergency department visits. The effects, however, are quite similar, as shown in Table 6.1.

Ancillary use has been reported in a variety of ways, including separate procedures, visits with laboratory or x-ray services, expenditures for laboratory or x-ray services, charges from freestanding laboratories, etc. As a result, it is not possible to make a fully informed estimate of the magnitude of reductions observed across the seven programs reporting results. Likewise, it is not possible to ascertain whether the reductions are due to reduced specialist contact, more concentration and coordination of care, or the reluctance of gatekeepers to prescribe marginally necessary tests. It is notable, however, that there is no evidence of the widespread increases in ancillary use that some observers suggested would occur if gatekeepers were to receive large numbers of new, unfamiliar patients. The findings, therefore, are consistent with Hypotheses 3 and 3a.

Observed reductions in prescription drug use were quite substantial. Reductions ranged from a low of 8 percent to highs of 20 to 30 percent. Increases in prescription drug use, where observed, were quite varied, ranging from less than 10 percent to 40 percent. One site reported rates doubling in one county and increasing by 50 percent in another, where family practice residents affiliated with a medical school provided services.

Inpatient use

The impact on inpatient use (as shown in Table 6.1) was much stronger and more pervasive than proposed by Hypotheses 4 and 4a. The only increase noted was for one site, which probably reflected differences in obstetrical stays for Medicaid-eligible enrollees. The range of inpatient reductions (see Table 6.3) was substantial.

It is necessary, however, to view these findings with caution. In most instances the analyses did not rigorously control for other factors that might have contributed to inpatient reductions. Most notably, Medicaid agencies added preadmission certification and other utilization review techniques concurrently with the introduction of PCCM programs. Thus, while the data support Hypotheses 4 and 4a, the attribution of these reductions exclusively to the gatekeeper intervention almost certainly overstates its impact.

Table 6.3 Reductions in Inpatient Use for 14 Programs

Programs Showing Reductions in Inpatient Use	*Percentage Reduction in Inpatient Use*
Wisconsin HMO Program	61
Nevada Enrolled Health Plan	>50
Michigan Medicaid Capitated Clinic Plan	50
Santa Barbara County (CA) Health Initiative	32 (children)
Colorado Primary Care Physician Program	>30
Oregon Medicaid Physician Care Organization Program	30 (3 counties)
Kitsap (WA) Sound Care Plan	10–30 (2 counties)
Michigan Medicaid Physician Sponsor Plan	25
Monterey County (CA) Health Initiative	17 (children)
Health Plan of San Mateo County (CA)	10
Minnesota Prepaid Medicaid Demonstration in Itasca County	8
Utah's Choice of Health Care Delivery Programs	7
HealthPASS of Philadelphia (PA)	1–7
Kansas Primary Care Network	2–3

Costs

Hypotheses 5 and 5a propose that small but significant reductions in Medicaid expenditures will be observed in the primary care gatekeeper programs.

The evidence as shown in Table 6.1 strongly supports the cost hypothesis, with approximately 80 percent of the programs reporting reductions in expenditures. For the two programs reporting cost increases, one had sharply increased payment rates to participating pediatricians as part of the demonstration intervention, leading to the overall increases in expenditures. In the other program the analysis established that because of a concurrent reduction in FFS expenditures in the comparison county, the basing of capitation rates on previous expenditure levels meant that the state actually paid more than it would have had the PCCM program not been implemented. This analysis is virtually the only one of its type performed, so it is not entirely comparable to the findings on costs from other programs. It is noteworthy that capitation rates were adjusted downward by over 15 percent in the following year to enable the state to realize savings.

It is difficult to simply and precisely estimate the size of cost reductions since the methods for computing savings varied so greatly, as discussed in Chapter 5. The net savings quoted ranged from lows of 1.5 percent and 3 percent to a high of 29 percent. Most states were in the 5 to 15 percent range. All the states with HMO or HIO contracts (with one exception) reported lower-than-expected expenditures (as further stated in Hypothesis 5), given the method for setting capitation rates. The actual amount of the savings for these programs is actually a function of savings per person and the number of enrolled beneficiaries, an issue that is discussed further in Chapter 7. This point underscores how less-intensive but easier-to-implement models of PCCM (e.g., with no risk-sharing) could produce absolute savings well in excess of more aggressive designs.

Subset of Programs with Stronger Assessments

In Chapter 5 we stated that, given the variability in program evaluation methods, it would be potentially misleading to give equal weight to the findings from each individual program. We therefore identified a subset of 12 programs deemed to have more reliable and valid assessments, to provide a more solid basis for assessing the impacts of PCCM on beneficiary use and cost experience. Table 6.4 includes the findings only from this subset of programs.

Table 6.4 Summary of Program Effects: Subset of 12 Programs with Stronger Assessments

	Increase	*Decrease*	*Mixed/ No Change*	*Unknown*
Physician visits	3 (25%)	5 (42%)	4 (33%)	0 (0%)
Emergency department use	0 (0%)	9 (75%)	0 (0%)	3 (25%)
Ancillary services	1 (8%)	7 (58%)	1 (8%)	3 (25%)
Prescription drug use	1 (8%)	5 (42%)	1 (8%)	5 (42%)
Inpatient use	1 (8%)	4 (33%)	5 (42%)	2 (17%)
Costs	2 (17%)	7 (58%)	2 (17%)	1 (8%)

Note: Numbers indicate the number of programs; percentages are a percent of all programs in that category. Percentages might not add up to 100 due to rounding.

The picture that emerges from looking at this subset is decidedly more conservative regarding the impact of gatekeeping. This view is most notable in three areas: physician visits, inpatient use, and costs. When results of the programs with weaker evaluations are removed, physician visits appear more likely to decrease. The reason for this decrease can be traced to the lack of sound evaluation in the omitted programs, which are mostly FFS gatekeeper programs. The higher level of physician use in these programs is not at all unreasonable given the use of FFS payments (plus a case management fee in many programs).

The inpatient effect is also more muted in the subset of reliably evaluated programs, since all the programs that were not included in the subset (with one exception) reported reduced inpatient use. This finding probably reflects the fact that the evaluations with the more rudimentary methodologies all attributed reductions in inpatient use to the PCCM intervention when in fact the reduction in inpatient use was pervasive across all payers and program models in the mid-1980s. The programs evaluated with stronger methods—typically person-level data with before and after and comparison group designs—were probably more successful in screening out this ''history'' effect (Cook and Campbell 1979).

We found a similar pattern when looking at cost effects because once again, virtually all programs reported cost savings. However, there are two additional explanations worth considering beyond the variation in methodological rigor in program assessments.

First, the source data for virtually all the omitted or less reliable programs (i.e., those not included in the subset) were waiver renewal applications which, as discussed earlier, had to demonstrate historical and expected future savings (i.e., cost-effectiveness) to receive HCFA approval for the waiver. Not surprisingly, every one of the 13 omitted programs reported savings. A more interesting issue pertaining to the more and the less reliable studies is that virtually all of the more reliable studies focused on the first years of program operations, while several of the omitted programs had a number of years of operational experience. Since there are virtually no rigorously conducted longitudinal studies of program effects on either cost or use, it is possible that more mature programs, like those omitted from the subset, could have larger or more certain savings. This point is discussed further in the final two chapters.

Use and Cost Effects by Design Features and Prototypes

Given the variation among the program designs in terms of both individual features and prototypes introduced in Chapter 4, it is useful to examine whether this variation is associated with differences in program effects. Initially, we examine the data by the design features of type of enrollment, organizational approach, and payment methods. The cost and use effects are then arrayed by the three program prototypes to assess whether there are discernable differences among them related to program outcomes.

Mandatory versus voluntary enrollment

There were six voluntary enrollment programs plus one program that was designed to be mandatory but was voluntary in practice during early implementation. We included this program with the mandatory programs. The summary of findings by type of enrollment is presented in Table 6.5.

The table suggests that there are no major differences between mandatory and voluntary programs, looking at the effects per person. Increases in physician visits appear more likely in the voluntary programs—possibly an indication of sick persons being more likely to join a voluntary program.

Voluntary programs also appear more likely to show an increase in inpatient use, but the numbers to support this expectation are few, allowing for only a qualitative interpretation. As suggested earlier, the major problem for voluntary programs has been in developing sufficiently large enrollments to make them viable and to justify the administrative expense. The six voluntary programs examined here had a total enrollment of less than 24,000, or on average fewer than 4,000 enrollees per program. Thus, per person savings do not necessarily translate into substantial aggregate savings.

Table 6.5 Summary of Program Effects: Mandatory versus Voluntary Enrollment

	Increase	*Decrease*	*Mixed/ No Change*	*Unknown*
Physician visits				
Mandatory programs	8 (42%)	7 (37%)	4 (21%)	0 (0%)
Voluntary programs	3 (50%)	1 (17%)	1 (17%)	1 (17%)
Emergency department use				
Mandatory programs	1 (5%)	10 (53%)	1 (5%)	7 (37%)
Voluntary programs	0 (0%)	3 (50%)	1 (17%)	2 (33%)
Ancillary services				
Mandatory programs	1 (5%)	6 (32%)	2 (11%)	10 (53%)
Voluntary programs	1 (17%)	1 (17%)	1 (17%)	3 (50%)
Prescription drug use				
Mandatory programs	2 (11%)	10 (53%)	1 (5%)	6 (32%)
Voluntary programs	1 (17%)	1 (17%)	1 (17%)	3 (50%)
Inpatient use				
Mandatory programs	0 (0%)	14 (74%)	4 (21%)	1 (5%)
Voluntary programs	1 (17%)	3 (50%)	1 (17%)	1 (17%)
Costs				
Mandatory programs	1 (5%)	15 (79%)	2 (11%)	1 (5%)
Voluntary programs	1 (17%)	4 (67%)	1 (17%)	0 (0%)

Note: Of the 25 programs in the study, 19 involved mandatory enrollment and 6 had voluntary enrollment. Numbers indicate the number of programs; percentages are the percent of all programs in that category. Percentages might not add up to 100 due to rounding.

State versus health insuring organization management

Seven of the 25 programs involved an HIO as a risk-assuming intermediary to develop and manage the PCCM program, while the remaining 18 used direct state administration. The findings in Table 6.6 show differences in program outcomes associated with organizational approach.

While impact differences between organizational approaches are not dramatic, they do suggest that HIO-managed programs might have had slightly stronger impacts on reducing (or not increasing) physician services, and in reducing inpatient use. The cost impact, as previously noted, displays a uniform reduction of costs to the state agency since HIOs contractually agree to provide care for a capitation rate based on a discount from expected FFS expenditures. It is not possible to discern, however, whether reductions in actual service expenditures accompanied payment by capitation.

Table 6.6 Summary of Program Effects: State versus Health Insuring Organization Management

	Increase	*Decrease*	*Mixed/ No Change*	*Unknown*
Physician visits				
State-run	9 (50%)	5 (28%)	3 (17%)	1 (6%)
HIO-run	2 (29%)	3 (43%)	2 (29%)	0 (0%)
Emergency department use				
State-run	0 (0%)	9 (50%)	2 (11%)	7 (39%)
HIO-run	1 (14%)	4 (57%)	0 (0%)	2 (29%)
Ancillary services				
State-run	2 (11%)	4 (22%)	2 (11%)	10 (56%)
HIO-run	0 (0%)	3 (43%)	1 (14%)	3 (43%)
Prescription drug use				
State-run	2 (11%)	7 (39%)	1 (6%)	8 (44%)
HIO-run	1 (14%)	4 (57%)	1 (14%)	1 (14%)
Inpatient use				
State-run	1 (6%)	11 (61%)	4 (22%)	2 (11%)
HIO-run	0 (0%)	6 (86%)	1 (14%)	0 (0%)
Costs				
State-run	2 (11%)	12 (67%)	3 (17%)	1 (6%)
HIO-run	0 (0%)	7 (100%)	0 (0%)	0 (0%)

Note: Of the 25 programs in the study, 18 were directly managed by the states and 7 were managed through HIOs. Numbers indicate the number of programs; percentages are the percent of all programs in that category. Percentages might not add up to 100 due to rounding.

Case manager method of payment: Fee-for-service versus capitation

We adapted the third program design feature, case manager method of payment, to permit a simplified contrast of FFS (with and without a case management fee) versus capitation made either to a PCP or primary care organization, or to a PHP. This departure from the original typology is necessary to offer a test of financial risk-sharing. This contrast leads into the contrast of the three prototypes, but combines Type 2 and Type 3 programs. The results of the contrast between capitation and FFS reimbursement are shown in Table 6.7.

The most notable difference among programs classified by reimbursement methodology is the greater likelihood that FFS programs will show increases in physician visits. There is also a slightly higher likelihood that prescription and ancillary use will be reduced in these programs. FFS programs are more likely to report differences in inpatient use, although the caveat noted above must again be recognized. There is virtually no difference in costs and emergency department use between FFS and capitated programs.

Program effects by program prototypes

Only three program features were selected for the separate analysis presented above since case manager selection and the scope of services are examined by implication in the following assessment by program prototype. We conclude the discussion of program findings by examining measures of use and cost effects by the three major program prototypes introduced in Chapter 4. The prototypes are restated as follows:

Type 1: FFS primary care gatekeeper enrollment

Type 2: At-risk primary care gatekeeper enrollment

Type 3: HMO or PHP enrollment

Table 6.7 Summary of Program Effects: Capitation versus Fee-for-Service Reimbursement

	Increase	*Decrease*	*Mixed/ No Change*	*Unknown*
Physician visits				
Capitation	6 (35%)	6 (35%)	4 (24%)	1 (6%)
FFS	5 (63%)	2 (25%)	1 (13%)	0 (0%)
Emergency department use				
Capitation	1 (6%)	9 (53%)	1 (6%)	6 (35%)
FFS	0 (0%)	4 (50%)	1 (13%)	3 (38%)
Ancillary services				
Capitation	2 (12%)	4 (24%)	2 (12%)	9 (53%)
FFS	0 (0%)	3 (38%)	1 (13%)	4 (50%)
Prescription drug use				
Capitation	2 (12%)	6 (35%)	4 (24%)	5 (29%)
FFS	1 (13%)	5 (63%)	0 (0%)	2 (25%)
Inpatient use				
Capitation	1 (6%)	10 (59%)	4 (24%)	2 (12%)
FFS	0 (0%)	7 (88%)	1 (13%)	0 (0%)
Costs				
Capitation	2 (12%)	14 (82%)	1 (6%)	0 (0%)
FFS	0 (0%)	5 (63%)	2 (25%)	1 (13%)

Note: Of the 25 programs in the study, 17 paid by capitation and 8 paid FFS. Numbers indicate the number of programs; percentages are the percent of all programs in that category. Percentages might not add up to 100 due to rounding.

Table 6.8 Summary of Program Effects: By Program Prototype and Overall

	Increase	*Decrease*	*Mixed/ No Change*	*Unknown*
Physician visits				
Type 1	5 (63%)	2 (25%)	1 (13%)	0 (0%)
Type 2	5 (45%)	3 (27%)	3 (27%)	0 (0%)
Type 3	1 (17%)	3 (50%)	1 (17%)	1 (17%)
Overall	11 (44%)	8 (32%)	5 (20%)	1 (4%)
Emergency department use				
Type 1	0 (0%)	4 (50%)	1 (13%)	3 (38%)
Type 2	1 (9%)	6 (55%)	0 (0%)	4 (36%)
Type 3	0 (0%)	3 (50%)	1 (17%)	2 (33%)
Overall	1 (4%)	13 (52%)	2 (8%)	9 (36%)
Ancillary services				
Type 1	0 (0%)	3 (38%)	1 (13%)	4 (50%)
Type 2	1 (9%)	3 (27%)	1 (9%)	6 (55%)
Type 3	1 (17%)	1 (17%)	1 (17%)	3 (50%)
Overall	2 (8%)	7 (28%)	3 (12%)	13 (52%)
Prescription drug use				
Type 1	1 (13%)	5 (63%)	0 (0%)	2 (25%)
Type 2	1 (9%)	5 (45%)	2 (18%)	3 (27%)
Type 3	1 (17%)	1 (17%)	0 (0%)	4 (67%)
Overall	3 (12%)	11 (44%)	2 (8%)	9 (36%)
Inpatient use				
Type 1	0 (0%)	7 (88%)	1 (13%)	0 (0%)
Type 2	0 (0%)	8 (73%)	2 (18%)	1 (9%)
Type 3	1 (17%)	2 (33%)	2 (33%)	1 (17%)
Overall	1 (4%)	17 (68%)	5 (20%)	2 (8%)
Costs				
Type 1	0 (0%)	5 (63%)	2 (25%)	1 (13%)
Type 2	1 (9%)	9 (82%)	1 (9%)	0 (0%)
Type 3	1 (17%)	5 (83%)	0 (0%)	0 (0%)
Overall	2 (8%)	19 (76%)	3 (12%)	1 (4%)

Note: There are 8 Type 1, 11 Type 2, and 6 Type 3 programs. Numbers indicate the number of programs; percentages are the percent of all programs in that category. Percentages might not add up to 100 due to rounding.

Table 6.8 presents program effects on cost and utilization by program prototype.

While Type 1 and Type 2 programs had similar patterns of generally increasing physician visits, the Type 3 PHPs were more likely to report reductions in physician visits. This difference could be due to under-reporting of physician visits; however, Type 2 programs that pay capitation for primary care services were also susceptible to underreporting and did not show the same pattern as Type 3 programs.

Virtually all programs were successful in reducing emergency department use. Essentially no differences were noted across the three program prototypes, as shown in the table. Also, no notable differences among the prototypes are detectable for ancillary use, other than the fact that data for this measure were less likely to be available from the Type 3 programs. As with ancillary use, Type 3 programs were less likely to report prescription use data, but overall the three prototypes had similar effects for prescription use.

Type 1 and Type 2 programs had similar effects for inpatient use. It is somewhat surprising that Type 3 programs appeared to lack strong effects for inpatient use, with one program reporting an increase and two reporting no change.

As previously stated, most programs reported reductions in cost, and there was no substantial difference in this variable among the three program types.

We conducted a final assessment to determine whether Type 2 programs had an internal difference based on whether the gatekeeper received capitation directly or whether an intermediary received the capitation and then disbursed payments to the gatekeepers. This analysis did not detect any systematic difference between these subtypes; thus, we concluded no need to subdivide Type 2 programs along this additional dimension.

Conclusion

We have analyzed the program effects presented in this chapter from several perspectives, including overall effects; effects from more reliable evaluation studies; effects based on program features; and finally, effects based on program prototypes. The next chapter presents the findings in more detail and delineates their implications for policy and management purposes.

References

Cook, T. D., and D. T. Campbell. 1979. *Quasi-Experimentation: Design and Analysis Issues for Field Settings.* Boston: Houghton-Mifflin.

Freund, D., L. Rossiter, P. Fox, J. Meyer, R. Hurley, T. Carey, and J. Paul. 1989. "Evaluation of the Medicaid Competition Demonstrations." *Health Care Financing Review* 11(2): 81–97.

Chapter 7

Discussion and Implications of the Evidence

The final two chapters address what is currently known and what is still unknown about Medicaid experience with PCCM. In this chapter we review and discuss our general findings. We reexamine and interpret variation based on critical structural features with regard to their policy implications. We present a discussion of the strengths and weaknesses of each of the three PCCM program prototypes. We also present our policy conclusions from the past decade of the diffusion of managed care in Medicaid. The limitations of the approach and our findings are reviewed in the final chapter, along with critical questions for future research.

Current Knowledge on the Effects on Use and Cost

After a decade of experience with a variety of models implementing PCCM for Medicaid, it is clear that these programs affect the utilization of health care services in a variety of categories. These programs also have detectable, although modest, effects on program cost to states and the federal government. It is not clear, however, how many of these effects are due to changes in *care-seeking* behavior by beneficiaries or to changes in *care-rendering* behavior by providers. In some instances, both behaviors might have been altered, and it would require considerable effort to disentangle the effects. Finally, some of the observed cost savings effects are solely due to contractual arrangements between state Medicaid agencies and HIO risk-assuming providers or intermediaries. It is unclear whether real resource use has changed under these models.

Emergency department use

The conceptual model we introduced in Chapter 2 suggested that two critical aspects are involved in primary care gatekeeping: (1) restriction on beneficiary choice of provider and (2) assumption by the provider of utilization management responsibilities. The fact that we consistently found sharp reductions in emergency department use for almost 80 percent of the programs included in our study provides an opportunity to illustrate this distinction. Beneficiaries are explicitly prohibited in all gatekeeper programs from seeking emergency department care for all but true emergencies. At the same time, they are formally enrolled with a gatekeeper as an alternative source of primary care services. Correspondingly, gatekeepers are contractually required to be available 24 hours a day either in person or through off-hour coverage arrangements. Moreover, the responsibility to preapprove nonemergency emergency department visits is lodged with gatekeepers as part of their utilization management responsibility. Several of the programs we reviewed included financial incentives or penalties to intensify the pressure on gatekeepers to manage access to the emergency department.

In general, the observed findings of lower emergency department use cannot be precisely attributed to changes in either beneficiary or provider behavior. However, in some of the programs there is useful related evidence. In Missouri's PHP (Type 3) program, two of the PHPs were hospital outpatient departments that used the emergency department for after-hour coverage. Evidence from these programs indicates weaker effects on emergency department use in these programs, suggesting that provider behavior had not necessarily changed but that beneficiaries did use the outpatient departments as an alternative site of care, at least during regular hours of operation. In Erie County, New York, the pediatric group that provided gatekeeper services used a children's hospital emergency department for its off-hour coverage and still reported a reduction in emergency department use of over 20 percent, suggesting that patients would alter their care-seeking away from the emergency department when a preferable alternative was available.

The overall emergency department findings are important because they suggest that care under PCCM is being sought and is subsequently received in less costly and, by most measures, more clinically desirable sites, given the impersonality and lack of continuity that characterizes most emergency department service delivery. Patients are receiving the benefits of primary care management as part of the primary care gatekeeping strategy.

The cost savings associated with the programs' effect on emergency department use, however, must be put into perspective. The volume of emergency department use, though problematic for Medicaid beneficiaries, still relates to only a relatively small proportion of beneficiaries—only 20 to 40 percent of the population use the emergency department in any given year, which translates into less than one-half visit per year per beneficiary. However, it is clearly a more serious problem in urban than in nonurban areas. For example, despite the 25 percent reduction in emergency department use, the rate of emergency department use at one urban site remained approximately four times as high as that found in the predominantly nonurban comparison counties. Thus, the proportionately large and widespread reductions in emergency department use observed in gatekeeper programs translate into only modest aggregate savings of Medicaid dollars. Additionally, many forgone emergency department visits are redirected to physician office visits. We still do not know whether having an identified PCP results in more telephone contact with a physician that might remove the need for either an emergency department visit or a physician office contact. Finally, where Medicaid programs have already introduced other strategies to reduce emergency department use—such as retrospective denial of payment for nonemergent care—then PCCM effects will be lessened.

Inpatient use

The programs reported reductions in inpatient use nearly as often as they reported reductions in emergency department visits. What is significant about these reductions is that while inpatient admissions are also infrequent, they are of disproportionately high cost; thus, even small decreases can produce substantial reductions in expenditures. Since physicians have always been de facto gatekeepers for hospital care, because only they have the legal authority to admit patients, the question of patient self-referral is not relevant. Reviewing the evidence leads to essentially a methodological question: To what extent can reductions in inpatient use under PCCM be attributed directly to gatekeepers' delegated utilization management activities?

It should be noted that we were unable to pose this question directly in the 25 studies we reviewed. We examined only those evaluations that attempted to control for or rule out other factors that could be contributing to what are the presumed PCCM effects. Before and after studies, for example, attempt to control for history or changes over time that are not related to the focal intervention. As suggested earlier, the period of time most of the programs examined, the mid-1980s, witnessed a proliferation of many inpatient utilization management techniques and presumably a resultant steady decline in inpatient utilization. There is widespread evidence that the long-term comparative advantage of HMOs versus indemnity plans in controlling inpatient use is now sharply diminished with the growth of managed care under the competing indemnity plans. Unless the evaluators' designs controlled for this trend, the changes they observed in inpatient use could be overstating the true impact of the PCCM intervention.

Our discussion in the previous chapter regarding the subset of studies we selected asserted that these programs' own findings were more conservative than those from the studies of lesser reliability. The subset studies were more likely to report no change or mixed findings in inpatient use, in part because their designs were more successful in isolating gatekeeper effects. Therefore, one must be cautious in arguing that PCCM leads with certainty to reductions in inpatient admissions.

Managed delivery systems that include a primary care gatekeeper nearly always include other features of utilization management that might be as effective or more effective than the gatekeeper feature. For example, the HealthPASS program in Philadelphia, which employs primary care gatekeeping, also has utilization review personnel on-site in hospitals to perform precertification and concurrent review. It might also be that individualized case management offered in a gatekeeper design improves the continuity of service, including more efficient preadmission care and better coordinated discharge planning, thereby reducing inpatient use. However, the main reason for an inpatient admission in the AFDC population is for obstetrical care. This area of care is subject to little discretionary change.

Physician visits

Our overall findings regarding physician visit effects tend to reinforce accepted tenets that incentives can affect the dynamics of gatekeeping. Despite the continuing problem of the underreporting of services covered under capitation payments, the evidence suggests that FFS gatekeeper programs lead to higher levels of physician visits. The capitated programs we examined reported either no change or lower levels of physician and related service contacts.

Unfortunately, the lack of precise measures in the programs' own studies masks interesting dynamics that can be explored for only a limited number of programs. Overall counts of physician visits are, in effect, net results of changes in both primary care and specialty care contacts. There is some evidence that primary care might be being substituted for specialty care, consistent with the hypotheses about the effects of PCCM. Once again, attributing this impact to either enrollee or gatekeeper behavior change, or to both, is problematic. For example, the restriction on the freedom of choice of provider prevents self-referral to a specialist. Therefore, one must expect some reduction of specialty care to accompany any gatekeeper program. In addition, channeling enrollees to primary care gatekeepers is expected to increase the proportion of care rendered by the PCPs. Finally, enlisting a gatekeeper to become the provider of first contact, and then offering incentives to reduce referral contacts, further increases the likelihood that fewer specialist visits will be observed.

Few studies have attempted to disentangle these effects. (Hurley, Freund, and Gage [1991] is an exception, as discussed below.) Therefore, overall, it appears that FFS gatekeeping is associated with more physician visits, while capitated (at-risk) gatekeeping is associated with no change in or fewer visits. It is likely that the substitution of primary for specialty care occurs in both arrangements. The difference observed might be because FFS arrangements encourage a compensating increase in primary care visits, which does not occur when the gatekeeper receives a fixed prepayment and residuals from referral or specialist care accounts. This issue has received less attention than it merits since, by implication, it illustrates the elasticity of the coordination or referral boundary between primary care and specialty physicians, as shown earlier in Figure 2.1. The implementation of the resource-based relative value scale (RBRVS) (Hsiao et al. 1988) is likely to provoke similar dynamics regarding the distribution of care provided by PCPs and specialty or referral physicians.

Other issues should be mentioned regarding potential changes in physician use under PCCM. First, if the health care system had impeded access before a gatekeeper program was implemented, the guaranteed availability of a regular source of care was likely to have resulted in more primary care visits (and more specialist visits as well), due to pent-up demand or the uncovering of treatable conditions. Second, when a program is introduced that permits individuals to have as their gatekeeper their prior primary care manager, it is possible that no change at all in use will be observed since business as usual (regarding care) is being maintained. Hurley, Freund, and Gage (1991) found this to be the case at two MCD sites where a significant proportion of the AFDC Medicaid eligibles were rollovers (i.e., they selected as their gatekeeper the physician or clinic they had as a regular source of care prior to the PCCM program). Finally, a large-scale dislocation of beneficiaries could lead to reduced use or, as reported in one program, a massive shifting of care from nonparticipating providers to providers willing to participate as gatekeepers.

Prescription and ancillary services use

Evidence on prescription and ancillary use under PCCM is equally, if not more, lacking in detail necessary to establish the findings as definitive. For example, changes in numbers of prescriptions tend to follow changes in counts of physician visits. However, the measures available from the programs do not indicate whether the prescribing behavior changed in either its clinical appropriateness or its cost-effectiveness. Concentrating more care with gatekeepers could reduce the possibility of unnecessary, redundant, or contraindicated prescriptions (because of drug interactions). It could also mean that less-costly drugs are prescribed, or that drugs typically seen as part of specialist care are not prescribed as often. There is virtually no literature on primary care gatekeeping and prescription behavior. The rough evidence of changes provides a starting point for more research in this area.

With respect to ancillary use, the major point is that enrollment with gatekeepers does not appear to be associated with any systematic increases in the use of ancillary services, defined as laboratory or x-ray services. It is plausible, but clearly not proven, that concentrating more care with a gatekeeper might result in small reductions in laboratory and x-ray workups. There is no evidence that usage increased as one might expect to see for workups of new patients if enrollment had disrupted prior physician-patient relationships. Further study on this question, as well as on the effects of including ancillary services within a primary care capitation payment, is needed.

Costs

Our review of the 25 primary care gatekeeping programs paints a convincing picture of the cost savings to state Medicaid agencies that can be expected. Our review also underscores that it is not easy to establish how large these savings are and how large they could be. Likewise, these savings are not always associated with reductions in resources consumed by Medicaid beneficiaries. They may be achieved solely at the expense of providers, plans, or intermediaries that agree to discounted rates for a variety of reasons. The reasons might vary from the desire to expand or maintain market share to believing that enhanced utilization management will more than offset the discounts from expected payments.

We found that the magnitude of savings, per beneficiary, is modest, typically in the 5 to 15 percent range. As discussed with regard to physician visits, the savings per beneficiary is a net effect of increases and decreases in various types of services. Decreases in emergency department use, although very substantial, represent only small reductions in cost per person. The mixed findings we have seen in physician visits suggest increases in expenditures in this category for many programs along with small reductions in others. Because many Medicaid programs use a fee schedule and do not pay a specialty differential, substitution effects might not produce direct cost savings for physician services. The reductions in inpatient care appear to be the source of most of the savings we observed, although they suggest larger savings than the programs actually are reporting, raising questions about the reliability of the reporting.

Increases in administrative costs due to PCCM program implementation have not been taken into account in many of the programs, particularly increases per beneficiary. This omission has the effect of further eroding estimated cost savings. On balance, however, the magnitude of marginal increases in costs due to administrative costs is rather small in the FFS programs, although case management fees can be substantial. In the programs that develop capitation rates and employ some type of individual beneficiary accounts, administrative efforts and expenses are proportionately higher and typically are borne by the state agency. Developing enrollee utilization and other monitoring management information systems is a major endeavor that has produced some of the most troublesome administrative problems for state agencies in both FFS and capitated gatekeeper programs. Contracting with HIOs or with HMOs or PHPs has provided an opportunity for states to shift some administrative costs to plans or intermediaries, making their administrative costs less comparable to those for the other types of programs. Overall, however, it should be noted that administrative cost data are rarely available and extremely difficult to disentangle. Moreover, comparability across programs and sites is not feasible due to different accounting conventions.

We have already mentioned the noncomparability of HMO and PHP estimates of cost savings. In these programs, the state has guaranteed savings by virtue of the negotiated, bid, or administered rates. Whether these savings are translated into less care or different types of care is virtually unknown at this point. Contractually guaranteed savings, along with the avoidance or shifting of administrative costs by the state, makes this strategy an appealing one.

A similar argument can be applied to programs that simply convert PCPs to FFS gatekeepers and pay them a case management fee, which is commonly interpreted as a long-overdue fee increase. The programs are administratively simple and highly acceptable to providers. The incremental costs, other than the case management fee and perhaps costs related to the production and dissemination of utilization reports, are relatively low. The fact that every one of these programs reports savings is notable, although not entirely persuasive.

Most of the remaining programs that use some form of risk-sharing, typically through paying a primary care capitation fee with some opportunity to participate in residuals in specialty/referral accounts, also claim savings. They are able to forgo the case management fee by offering opportunities for intensified gatekeeper utilization management that allow for bonuses from the year-end risk pool. On the other hand, these programs incur higher administrative costs (and often provider resistance) in the process of developing rates and maintaining the data necessary to account for and settle residual accounts. In effect, they are counting on financial incentives to motivate reductions necessary to make participation profitable or, at least, acceptable. It must be noted, however, that with the exception of reductions in physician visits, there is no strong evidence to suggest that utilization is more rigorously managed in these programs than under FFS gatekeeper programs.

The foregoing discussion largely endorses the idea that there is more than one way to realize the savings Medicaid administrators are seeking. However, because there have been no sound assessments of long-term cost effects for any of these gatekeeping programs, a definitive test of cost savings is not available. Supporters of capitation or risk-based payments have long argued that they build in an incentive for continuous improvement to outperform the capitation rates. It must be noted, however, that the history of low payments in Medicaid raises serious questions about just how much continuous improvement in performance can be expected. On the other hand, supporters of FFS primary care management contend that this approach will achieve its desired effects if it is sucessful in recruiting as gatekeepers efficient providers of care.

A final but important consideration in terms of examining cost savings in PCCM programs must be the size of the enrollment base of the program. In an interesting analysis reported in the MPE, the authors showed achieved savings in the six programs and then projected these savings into the future based on maximum enrollment of all covered groups in the program (ORD 1987). Not surprisingly, they demonstrated that programs that enroll a large number of beneficiaries, even with small per person savings, could produce substantial reductions in aggregate Medicaid expenditures. The implication of their analysis is that programs that have high administrative feasibility, garner widespread provider support, and can be expeditiously implemented will produce large aggregate savings—even when their impact per person is relatively small. Thus, a state such as Kentucky, with nearly 200,000 beneficiaries in a low-intensity FFS gatekeeper program, can realize aggregate savings well in excess of the savings demonstrated by programs with more elegant risk-sharing schemes but with substantially lower levels of provider and beneficiary participation.

Significance of Program Design Features

One of the major goals of this study has been to examine how specific features of program design are associated with program outcomes. Our findings in this regard are summarized below.

Mandatory versus voluntary enrollment

The data we presented in Chapter 6 suggested that program effects did not differ substantially based on voluntary versus mandatory enrollment, particularly when we looked at person-level data. However, the voluntary programs we examined were dramatically smaller than the mandatory programs; thus the changes detected do not have major financial importance for the state Medicaid agencies that implemented them. The problem of inducing beneficiaries to voluntarily select managed care arrangements has persisted since well before the introduction of the post-OBRA PCCM programs studied here. Most HMOs have not enhanced the relatively comprehensive basic Medicaid benefits, especially given the capitation rate Medicaid agencies are willing to pay. While primary care might, in principle, be more readily accessible to beneficiaries who select an HMO, the various mechanisms to manage care probably do not make it appear as accessible in practice to potential enrollees.

It is also possible that the apparent savings in voluntary HMOs are a result of favorable selection, as suggested in the RAND evaluation of the Robert Wood Johnson Foundation–supported initiatives (Buchanan et al. 1992). This study of the experience of one hospital-based HMO found substantial differences in use and expenditures between self-selectors into the HMO and random assignees into the HMO. Self-selectors into FFS and random assignees to FFS both had levels of cost and use nearly identical to those for persons randomly assigned to the HMO. However, the researchers issued two important caveats related to their study. First, the findings were based on the experience of a single, distinctive, hospital-based HMO with an enrollment of only approximately 2,000 Medicaid beneficiaries, from which it might be difficult to generalize. Second, they noted that the analysis of a different plan, which led to different conclusions, was not included in the preliminary study. To reiterate, it is highly unlikely that voluntary enrollment in HMOs can offer opportunities for substantial cost savings in Medicaid.

State versus health insuring organization program management

Given current legislative restrictions on new HIOs, the question of their preferability to state administration has been reduced to a moot point. Furthermore, the evidence presented by the programs' evaluations is not conclusive regarding the use of HIOs except for the fact that contracting with HIOs guarantees reductions in expected Medicaid expenditures for the state agency. Risk-shifting to the HIO has proven to be manageable in most instances, although the failure of one early HIO program is certainly a notable exception (Aved 1987). On the other hand, relationships between states and HIOs have had to weather a large of amount of controversy and dispute, primarily over rate negotiation (Anderson and Fox 1987). The cost-and-use focus of this book also does not permit a commentary on how well one of the asserted HIO advantages—local customization of the Medicaid program—has worked. This aspect, however, might have significant implications in terms of garnering provider support and overcoming provider and beneficiary resistance.

Case manager selection and qualification

The range of qualifications necessary for providers to participate in the 25 programs varies from individual, licensed PCPs to exclusively preexisting HMOs. Selection and qualification decisions are associated with the goals for the program, such as directly linking beneficiaries with a PCP or integrating them into established PHPs. They are also associated with provider supply and capacity and with states having to accommodate these constraints when assessing provider availability and likely participation. Furthermore, they are affected by the willingness of local provider communities to accept innovative approaches to either salvage or enhance a Medicaid program perhaps in need of fundamental change. Finally, they might be driven by the basic assumptions of program developers about what critical problems exist in the current Medicaid program (e.g., access, cost, quality) and what type of case manager participation will be most responsive to these problems.

The overwhelming impression we obtained by observing the variety in program designs on this feature is that the approach must fit local market conditions. For example, in many urban areas there are virtually no individual or even small groups of PHPs. Most providers are affiliated with hospitals or health centers. Thus, the idealized view of individual physician case managers must give way in reality to major adaptations. For this reason, there are examples of health centers or hospitals participating as case-managing entities, often as PHPs capitated for all or a portion of covered services. This arrangement might appear to be simply a conversion of conventional Medicaid providers from FFS to prepayment, and in some instances that has been the case. However, there are also notable examples, such as in Michigan, Missouri, and Philadelphia, where large, publicly supported facilities have availed themselves of the opportunity to make the transition to bona fide managed-care PHPs.

Is PCCM fully articulated and practiced in all of the 25 programs? Simply stated, it is not. Virtually all programs that are still operational do have specifications for gatekeeper performance, with the possible exception of some of the PHPs that do not subscribe to the usefulness of individualized primary care gatekeeping. However, some programs with physician-specific performance requirements do not observe them fully, and thus allow organizations to act as gatekeepers. In some respects, this arrangement might undermine the merits of individualized care management, although the data generally are not sufficiently detailed to measure compliance with performance requirements.

On the other hand, questions can be raised about the appropriateness of purchasers of care attempting to micromanage service delivery within managed care plans. Contracting with organizations for a full scope of services, rather than with individual physicians for the provision, brokering, and authorization of services, is a common practice that has the effect of shifting the burden to the subcontracting organization for directly monitoring physician performance. The monitoring of physician performance then becomes part of the service being purchased and can make the organization a more reliable and potentially accountable entity with which to contract than an individual physician would be. Thus, the scope of service being obtained from the case manager is intertwined with the type of case manager (individual physician or organization) with whom the purchaser is contracting.

Case management methods of payment

As stated earlier, current evidence does not permit us to conclude that risk-based (e.g., capitation) methods of payment have a material effect on cost and use, beyond the distinctive exception of physician visits. There are several plausible explanations for this finding beyond just the limited availability of data. It is possible that the incentives that have been used are relatively weak. The incentives might also be so complex that providers cannot respond to them and alter their behavior accordingly. In other instances, risk-based payments to organizations such as HMOs do not translate into direct at-risk experience for employed or contracted physicians. A further possibility is that incentives are important only after a large number of patients in any practice are covered. While it is not known what the threshold number of patients is, it might be larger than the number we encountered in most of the observed programs.

Two other distinctively Medicaid-related possibilities about why no effects were found should be mentioned. The types and volumes of care rendered to Medicaid beneficiaries might not be amenable to substantial change, or at least to change that could somehow be influenced by payment methods, such as care related to pregnancy and childbirth. A second point is that the decision of providers to participate or continue to participate in Medicaid after years of low payment rates is not exclusively, or even predominately, economic. These providers might have largely given up on the potential profitability of Medicaid patients. To expect providers now to see Medicaid beneficiaries in more purely economic terms, given only marginal potential revenue gains, might be unrealistic.

Finally, the evidence that we examined regarding FFS with case management fees leads to an important finding that needs to be reiterated. The fact that five of the eight programs in this study paying in this manner experienced increases in physician visits, and one other had no change, strongly suggests that this variety of PCCM has not inhibited access to care but in fact has demonstrably improved it. As more Medicaid programs look to primary care management as a cost-saving strategy, this finding is likely to gain greater importance because it counteracts concerns about reduced access due to restriction on freedom of choice.

Pros and Cons of the Program Prototypes

We initially derived and described the three prototypes to enable us to aggregate use and cost findings into reasonably homogeneous categories of programs and to investigate whether there were outcome differences among them. We found that the outcome differences were relatively limited, except for the increase in physician visits noted for Type 1 programs. This lack of difference suggests that Medicaid managers can achieve modest savings in various ways. Since one of the hallmarks of Medicaid has been its variation across states, this finding is not surprising. It is instructive, however, to discuss the advantages of each of the three prototypical programs over the others, in terms of the possible context, expectations, and goals of program developers.

Type 1 programs

The appeal of the FFS primary care gatekeeper enrollment model is strongest in terms of its administrative simplicity and its potential for minimal disruption of both existing delivery systems and of established physician-patient relationships. The disruption of existing relationships is seen as directly counter to promoting stability and continuity in care. The Type 1 interventions have encountered less provider resistance than the other two prototypes, and case management fees, where implemented, can be viewed positively as a long-overdue fee augmentation.

The unobtrusiveness of the design and minimal disruption of patients from prior usual sources of care also avoids potential patient dissatisfaction and its accompanying problems. The fact that gatekeepers do not participate in savings from reduced referral care avoids engendering hostility from specialists, and, in most instances, gatekeepers maintain the same referral network previously in place. The 24-hour availability requirement has not proven onerous to providers, since it is compatible with normal professional responsibility. Additionally, assured access to care (and the evidence that it has an impact on the level of physician visits) has considerable appeal to policymakers sensitive to criticism that gatekeeping is a pernicious, if not punitive, strategy. The evidence from Type 1 programs directly contradicts such criticism. Finally, these types of programs have greatly expanded in size in relatively short periods of time.

Persistent concerns about Type 1 programs include that they are too much "business as usual" and fail to provide incentives to physicians to practice gatekeeping vigorously. Early Type 1 programs were weak in the specification of gatekeeper duties and not at all selective in who qualified for this role. There was also concern that promoting affiliation with a provider would result in overutilization because self-limiting diseases would now be uncovered and unnecessarily treated. There was also the concern that a lack of incentives to curb referral care would result in increases rather than decreases in this area. To compensate for the lack of financial incentives, monitoring mechanisms would have to be introduced. These mechanisms could be difficult to design, implement, and disseminate and could result in unpopular provider sanctions or exclusions based on poor performance. In other words, the apparent administrative simplicity of this design could give way to increased costs and difficulty to properly monitor it.

If the savings reported from Type 1 programs can be accepted—the evidence, as noted above, is not entirely conclusive—they must be judged as largely successful. Moreover, they seem to be striking the desired balance between cost control and access enhancement, or more precisely cost control via access enhancement. The principal limitation of this conclusion is that all these programs are probably overstating or at least overattributing inpatient reductions to the impact of gatekeeping. However, these are not the only reductions noted, so cost decreases retain credibility. The Type 1 programs clearly are the simplest programs to introduce and to expand quickly to large populations. Thus, they can deliver relatively substantial savings, although the savings lack the predictability that fixed, prepaid rates guarantee.

Type 2 programs

These programs represent nearly half of the PCCM initiatives we studied. They also represent a more heterogeneous mix of programs than the other two prototypes. This heterogeneity contributes to a mixed outcome experience, as discussed earlier. The major distinction in these at-risk primary care gatekeeping programs is that they seek incentives to influence gatekeepers to use resources more carefully. This more careful use might mean rationing primary care or using referral sources more judiciously.

By assuming that the behavior of the PCP is financially motivated, these programs offer inducements in the form of improved cash flow via capitation and opportunities to share in residuals in individual or pooled referral accounts. At the same time, many of the designs attempt to allow doctor-patient relationships to be sustained and to promote individualized case management as offered in Type 1 programs.

Assuming that current providers will accept at-risk (capitation) payment, continuity can be maintained and promoted. In response to incentives, primary care gatekeepers are expected to concentrate more care with themselves and perhaps expand the scope of conditions treated or the intensity of services directly rendered. This would include making themselves more available to prevent unnecessary emergency department visits. Similarly, promoters of capitation have long asserted that more preventive care will be rendered to enrollees if the providers have incentives to treat conditions before more costly sequelae develop. Finally, utilization monitoring and performance feedback systems are needed to support case management and to assist at-risk gatekeepers in clinical decision making. Several of these features are consistent with systems that are growing in popularity in private sector managed care programs. Thus, Medicaid can use Type 2 program designs to dovetail its efforts with private sector developments. Finally, prepayment through capitation implies predictability in expenditures. State Medicaid agencies have sought, through Type 2 programs, to gain at least a modicum of predictability through primary care capitation payments.

The problems associated with the promotion of Type 2 programs are also important, however. The single most important problem is achieving adequate provider participation in a risk-sharing relationship with a potentially unreliable partner—the so-called public sector risk factor that has plagued the Medicare HMO-risk contract program (Bell 1987). Many providers simply do not see the risk they are assuming as offset by a reasonable expectation of gain. This perception might be because rates are seen as too low or because they question the ability of the state agencies to manage these programs effectively and equitably. The immediate consequence of fewer participating providers is that existing relationships are certain to be disrupted. Disruption in turn engenders dissatisfaction among both providers and beneficiaries. Massive shifting in sites of care, as happened in the Citicare program, can also occur when providers who chose to participate are not the traditional sources of care for the Medicaid-eligible population (Freund 1984).

Further problems arise in the rate setting or rate negotiation process. This process is often a complex enterprise, and there might be little experience or expertise on which to draw within the Medicaid agencies. It also means the programs must begin new data collection and data analysis efforts and develop new monitoring and reporting systems. Furthermore, to counteract some of the direct risk-sharing problems, they must develop stop-loss arrangements or, alternatively, create pools of physicians to reduce the risk to individual physicians of uncontrollable or unexpectedly high enrollee expenses. All these accommodations are administratively demanding and represent additional points of disagreement that must be resolved to achieve an acceptable level of provider participation.

In light of the additional demands associated with the Type 2 programs, we must ask the question: Does the evidence support the contention that risk-sharing or capitation is worth the attendant problems? The answer seems to be no, although the level of detail in most of the programs' analyses to date precludes a definitive conclusion. Physician visits are lower in these programs versus Type 1 programs, but this result might be an artifact of the underreporting of capitated services. On every other measure of use and costs, there is virtually no difference between the two types of programs. This finding is important and clearly demands further scrutiny and challenge. Moreover, this finding for Type 1 programs parallels the experience of PPOs in the private sector. Most PPOs have avoided using risk-sharing methods of payment but appear (or at least claim) to generate cost savings equal to those of HMOs even in the absence of risk-sharing at the physician level.

Type 3 programs

Medicaid agencies have attempted to enroll beneficiaries in established HMOs and other PHPs for more than 15 years. This effort has not been especially successful, with only about 5 percent of all beneficiaries enrolled, compared to a population-wide HMO penetration rate of 15 percent (GHAA 1992). Fewer than 25 of the nearly 550 HMOs nationwide have Medicaid enrollments in excess of 15,000 members (HCFA 1991). These data largely testify to the failure of the promotion of voluntary HMO enrollment for the reasons discussed earlier. With the exception of the special case of Arizona, only two states, Ohio and Wisconsin, have attempted to mandate enrollment exclusively in HMOs, and they have done so in only two cities.

Why has Medicaid persisted in these efforts to promote HMO enrollment? In part, to gain the benefits of the well-established managed-care system. Chief among these benefits have been the reductions in inpatient use that have been synonymous with HMOs for nearly two decades. The predictability of capitation payments for virtually the entire Medicaid benefit package is highly appealing to policymakers, especially if these payments can be achieved through competitive bidding, like in Arizona, or through aggressive negotiation, as in other states. In addition, as HMOs grew rapidly in the 1980s, enrollment in them was viewed as an opportunity for Medicaid beneficiaries to gain access to mainstream providers. By definition, HMOs represent comprehensive delivery systems, including organized and accountable providers inculcated (in theory, at least) with the values of primary care management and the promotion of preventive services.

The negative aspects of HMO and PHP enrollment from the state agency standpoint again include potential disruption of established doctor-patient relationships. Intermittent eligibility, which is characteristic of the Medicaid population, presents both logistical and financial obstacles to enrolling persons in a system of care that requires predictability in expenditures to set adequate rates. The organized and regimented delivery systems found in HMOs can also be challenging to culturally or educationally disadvantaged beneficiaries, thus presenting a potential threat to access for these persons (Ware et al. 1986). In addition, the preponderance of women needing obstetrical care in the eligible population has meant that HMOs are understandably reluctant to enroll persons who will incur initial expenses well in excess of a monthly capitation rate. As the Washington Group Health Cooperative (GHC) study illustrates, this problem is compounded when eligibility ends before initial losses can be covered. This situation is really a special case of selection bias that was unfavorable to the GHC plan. Favorable selection to the plans can also occur, in which Medicaid programs end up paying more for HMO enrollment of beneficiaries than they would have paid if the individuals had remained in the FFS sector.

Trying to do business with well-established HMOs has been problematic for impoverished state Medicaid programs, especially during periods of rapid growth in private sector enrollees for the HMOs. Medicaid agencies that have set their rates on a low FFS equivalent base have found far fewer interested HMOs than they hoped for. The public sector risk factor issue enters again when HMOs fear that rates might be excessively or prematurely ratcheted down if they achieve a margin of success (Riley, Coburn, and Kilbreth 1990). This concern is compounded by the state agencies' lack of experience in managing care for this population, which can challenge existing service delivery and control systems. As an alternative to dealing only with established HMOs, specially waivered Medicaid-only PHPs have been established to meet unmet demand. While some of these programs have proven to be very successful, others have experienced financial and other problems that challenge the stability and credibility of the HMO and PHP enrollment strategy. Finally, Medicaid agencies have had a lot to learn about contract negotiation and performance monitoring with HMOs. The oversight of services provided by these organizations needs to be decidedly different from the traditional, case-by-case and highly uneven provider oversight performed for the FFS Medicaid sector.

The evidence we have presented here for Type 3 programs is selective in that it includes only six sites and represents mixed results except in terms of cost savings. The nature of the contracting process virtually guarantees savings when rates are set based on a discount from FFS. If a sufficiently large enrollment can be achieved, as in the mandatory programs, then very large savings are possible and the promotion of this strategy is clearly justified. However, this point underscores the limited applicability of this strategy since there are relatively few locations in the country where mandatory programs of this magnitude seem feasible. Combining this point with (1) rapid change in the HMO industry, (2) growing competition from other forms of managed care entities, and (3) the consolidation among existing plans, there is reason for skepticism that this strategy will prove a fruitful one for most Medicaid programs. However, it would be possible for HMO enrollment to receive a boost if more states were to adopt statewide Type 1 programs that permit beneficiaries the option of HMOs as well as PCCM gatekeepers.

Critical Conclusions from a Decade of Primary Care Case Management Experience

This chapter has discussed the implications of our findings with regard to PCCM in Medicaid. We conclude by identifying a series of observations regarding the past decade of the diffusion of these types of programs. The conclusions represent our views based on the evidence presented here, as well as our (and others') collective experience studying the phenomenon. Although our study is the most extensive review of evidence yet undertaken, it has a number of limitations that we summarize in the final chapter. Most significantly, however, we have examined only structural features and cost and use outcomes. Many other aspects of these programs are also important, such as patient satisfaction, provider participation, and quality of care. These aspects are worthy of the same degree of attention as we have given to cost and use effects. Chapter 8 also presents a series of unanswered but critical questions as areas for future research.

Concluding statements regarding PCCM are as follows:

PCCM has survived an uneven first decade in terms of its performance; however, it is likely to grow substantially in the next decade. It has produced modest savings and has altered patterns of use in detectable and desirable ways. Growth in the future will benefit from private sector expansion of managed care arrangements that will reinforce Medicaid's embracing of managed care. Budgetary pressures will compel more states to seek strategies that have proven records of nearly certain (albeit modest) savings.

Most of the criticism and concern voiced regarding restricting freedom of choice of provider have not been justified based on the past decade of PCCM experience. States seem to be having success in finding adequate numbers of desirable providers to participate as gatekeepers. The evidence of use effects suggests that either (1) major changes in delivery patterns have not occurred or (2) those that have occurred, such as reduced emergency department use, are generally viewed as positive. Though we have not explicitly addressed quality of care, we found no evidence in any of the 25 programs of reductions in quality of care from that provided by FFS Medicaid. Finally, the very concept of freedom of choice of provider is undergoing major redefinition as managed care models are replacing the indemnity insurance system for medical care across the board.

The PCCM strategy appears to have effectively improved access to primary care for Medicaid beneficiaries. Every one of the 1.2 million beneficiaries in these 25 programs has, by design, a contractually obligated regular source of care who must be available 24 hours a day, seven days a week. This statement is a powerful commentary on the success of these programs and constitutes a critical difference between these Medicaid recipients and many of their fellow beneficiaries remaining in the conventional FFS Medicaid program.

The variety in program designs we observed in this study suggests that there is no one best way to obtain the benefits of PCCM. Program designers must factor in many issues and attempt to meet a complex set of competing goals. Outcome evidence alone is not sufficiently prescriptive to allow policymakers to endorse one program type over another. Administrative feasibility and the magnitude of potential beneficiary enrollment offer critical guidance to prospective program developers.

As the number and types of alternative utilization management techniques grow, it will become increasingly difficult for program evaluators to persuasively attribute savings and other effects to the gatekeeper intervention alone. The entire medical marketplace in the United States is in transition, for private and public beneficiaries alike. As private sector programs intensify their cost-management efforts, the distinctions between Medicaid and these other programs are likely to diminish. This development is likely to increase mutual and reciprocal learning between the sectors.

The contribution of prepayment and risk-sharing in general is inconclusive in the Medicaid PCCM experience. We have not been able to demonstrate the capacity of capitation to shape and control use patterns. However, the appeal to administrators of predictability in specifying at least short-term expenditures is unquestionable, particularly in an era of diminishing state budgets. Instability in the prepaid HMO market, and in the health insurance industry as a whole, raises questions and concerns about whether risk-based products will survive their many contemporary challenges. Medicaid's implicit status as a self-insured preferred provider network should be recognized as a possible model for many future private sector initiatives.

Embedded in the dynamics of primary care gatekeeping are some potentially illuminating lessons about future relationships between PCPs and specialists. These relationships are also in transition, and more conflict and contention must be expected, especially in light of the pending implementation of the RBRVS for Medicare. If anticipated shifts in supply and income for PCPs ensue as a result of RBRVS, then Medicaid could experience both reinforcement and expansion in its efforts to develop primary care gatekeeping programs.

The quality of evaluation evidence from the first decade of experience with PCCM in Medicaid is mixed. The many limitations of the programs' own evaluations probably have led to unrealistic and unsubstantiated claims about the cost savings potential. Alternatively, what has been learned has not been effectively disseminated to guide policymakers and program developers nearly as well as it could be. The proverbial wheel has been reinvented many times over, and confusion and suspicion about the desirability of the PCCM strategy has persisted.

The lack of definitive evidence has also been confusing to both participating and prospective providers. As private sector managed care initiatives grow, acceptance in the provider community of Medicaid initiatives should also grow, although private sector–based evidence has also had many limitations. The major impediments for Medicaid will remain its reputation as the most penurious of payers, the concern that it will always opt for cost savings over other concerns, and its perceived penchant for cost shirking. It is not yet clear to providers whether Medicaid administrators have learned the one great lesson of their program—you don't get something if you're not willing to pay for it.

Much of the source data for our analysis has come from waiver renewal applications and their accompanying supporting documentation. Many of these documents are not of high quality and are nearly perfunctory in their assertion of savings. They read much like certificate of need applications of the 1970s and 1980s and, also like these applications, have apparently received perfunctory reviews. Also, state Medicaid personnel generally see the waiver process as a burdensome ritual and, based on the quality of evidence presented, typically not worthy of serious analytical effort. At the policy level, waiver reform ought to consider either intensifying the expectations for such submittals or, alternatively, adopting a less burdensome process to continue programs that initially attain satisfactory credibility and stature.

References

Anderson, M., and P. Fox. 1987. "Lessons Learned from Medicaid Managed Care Approaches." *Health Affairs* 6(1): 71–86.

Aved, B. 1987. "The Monterey County Health Initiative: A Post-Mortem Analysis of a California Demonstration Project." *Medical Care* 25(1): 35–45.

Bell, C. 1987. "Fallon Community Health Plan, A Medicare Experience." In *Hospital-Sponsored HMOs*, ed. G. J. Rahn. Chicago: American Hospital Association.

Buchanan, J., A. Leibowitz, J. Keesey, J. Mann, and C. Damberg. 1992. *Cost and Use of Capitated Medical Services: Evaluation of the Program for Prepaid Managed Health Care*. RAND/UCLA/Harvard Center for Health Care Financing Policy Research. Santa Monica, CA: RAND Corporation.

Group Health Association of America (GHAA). 1992. *National Directory of HMOs*. Washington, DC: The Association.

Freund, D. 1984. *Medicaid Reform: Four Studies of Case Management*. Washington, DC: American Enterprise Institute.

Health Care Financing Administration (HCFA). 1991. *Medicaid Coordinated Care Enrollment Report*. Baltimore, MD: Medicaid Bureau, HCFA.

Hsiao, W. C., P. Braun, D. Yntema, and E. R. Becker. 1988. "Estimating Physicians' Work for a Resource-Based Relative Value Scale." *New England Journal of Medicine* 319(13): 835–41. See also commentary in same issue by William Roper, M.D., pp. 865–67.

Hurley, R. E., D. Freund, and B. Gage. 1991. "Gatekeeper Effects on Patterns of Physician Use." *Journal of Family Practice* 32(2): 167–74.

Office of Research and Demonstrations (ORD). 1987. *Medicaid Program Evaluation: Final Report*. Report No. MPE 9.2. Eds. J. Holahan, J. Bell, and G. S. Adler. Baltimore, MD: HCFA.

Riley, P., A. Coburn, and E. Kilbreth. 1990. *Medicaid Managed Care: The State of the Art—A Guide for States*. Portland, ME: National Academy for State Health Policy and the Edmund S. Muskie Institute of Public Affairs, University of Southern Maine.

Ware, J., R. Brooks, W. Rogers, E. Keeler, A. Davies, C. Sherburne, G. Goldberg, P. Camp, and J. Newhouse. 1986. "Comparison of Health Outcomes at a Health Maintanence Organization with Those of Fee-for-Service." *Lancet* (8488): 1017–22.

Chapter 8

Addressing the Unknowns: Study Limitations and Areas for Future Research

We noted earlier that public policy evaluation by its very nature is a complex, costly, and, at times, contentious enterprise. None of the many evaluations of Medicaid PCCM programs has avoided these challenges. In investigating all of these studies, we faced a number of limitations that must be acknowledged. At the same time, our effort to make sense of this material gave us an opportunity to identify and enumerate many unaddressed or unanswered questions about use and cost effects under PCCM.

This chapter begins with a review of our study's limitations. It then examines a number of important methodological issues that future research and evaluation initiatives will have to address. Finally, it identifies a series of specific areas that merit additional investigation to answer critical remaining questions about PCCM in Medicaid.

Limitations of the Study

Given the substantial number of studies from which we could have acquired and collated data, a meta-analytic approach (Hunter, Schmidt, and Jackson 1982; Light and Pillemer 1984) would have seemed the ideal approach with which to address these findings. However, meta-analysis presupposes a well-defined phenomenon and randomized designs. This is clearly not the case for this study, given the heterogeneity found in PCCM programs in Medicaid. Thus we had to develop, as a starting point, a framework for classifying and then grouping the programs to organize the findings in a manageable and interpretable fashion. The consequence of this approach is that we had to make major assumptions about program similarities to accomplish the synthesis. The potential arbitrariness of these assumptions is a key and fundamental limitation of the study.

Moreover, even within the prototypes we designated, we noted substantial differences among the programs. In addition, our characterization of all three types as different variations of primary care gatekeeping can be challenged. For example, enrollment in HMOs that do not explicitly assign enrollees to individual physicians implies that organizations can be gatekeepers, which is not wholly compatible with the basic philosophy of providing individual, primary care management to every beneficiary. Nonetheless, the program prototypes appear to have reasonable within-group coherence and comparability.

Great variation exists in the quality of the data we reviewed. It can be asserted that program impact projections that are developed internally are not comparable to, or cannot be combined with, some of the sophisticated and elegant evaluations conducted for other programs. The RAND (Buchanan et al. 1992) and Suffolk County (Hohlen et al. 1990) evaluations are probably the closest to ideal designs among the studies we included. By relying on unpublished sources for many of our findings, we placed an added onus on ourselves to appraise the validity and reliability of the programs' evaluation findings. Although we invested significant effort in this appraisal, there appears throughout our study the usual tension between rigor and relevance. In most cases we have chosen to include as much of the evidence as possible. Readers ultimately must decide whether to accept the preponderance of both definitive and illustrative evidence or to more modestly and cautiously limit their conclusions to those supported by the more rigorously conducted evaluations. A serious complication of accepting only the best supported conclusions, however, is that few Type 1 programs have had high-quality appraisals. Since these programs have considerable appeal because of the size of their potential enrollment and their ease of implementation, they appear to have much to recommend them. Nevertheless, the lack of persuasive evaluation evidence clearly has to qualify any endorsement of them.

When Hurley and Freund first published their typology of Medicaid managed care (1988), a reviewer noted that a crucial missing feature of their classification scheme was the political or administrative context of a program. Two dimensions of this criticism merit mention here. First, for our study of 25 programs, we avoided reporting much of the published evidence in case studies that described delays and slippage in program development, as well as design and implementation problems, which obviously are directly and indirectly associated with program outcomes. Second, we do not address the local (including state) climates into which these programs were introduced, which undoubtedly influence such key considerations as program acceptability to providers and beneficiaries. In addition, the quality and condition of the conventional FFS Medicaid program when the new initiatives were introduced clearly affects the willingness of program participants to accept or resist innovation. Omitting these and other hard-to-classify background features means that our model does not capture a great deal of unexplained variation, because it contains, by necessity, only a limited set of all possible structural variables and factors.

A special case of this limitation is the fact that most of the better evaluations included in this study were based on the early years of the programs when they might not have reached a steady state. Because many of the programs were demonstrations or pilot programs, both providers and beneficiaries might have been tentative and skeptical about the programs' durability and longevity. Alternatively, the new programs could have experienced a favorable Hawthorne effect with unsustainably high resource investments that ultimately faded as the programs became routinized. Finally, program design changes to correct problems or accommodate obstacles cannot be captured in static or cross-sectional analyses. We could do little to address, let alone correct, this limitation for our study, since we relied on evaluations already completed.

The focus of our study has been on program structure and its relationship to a limited number of cost and use outcome measures. While *focus* connotes clarity, it also implies narrowness. We have ignored many important aspects of program outcomes in this study. One reason was the need to restrict the examined issues and thereby ensure the manageability of the study. The maximum number of programs systematically examined in any previous study was six, in both the Medicaid Competition Demonstrations and the Medicaid Program Evaluation. Because we were able to use a sample size four times larger, the approach we preferred for our study was to review a relatively small set of outcome measures that we believed to be available in most of the selected programs. The price of this parsimony is a less-than-complete picture of how the programs worked in other critical areas such as access to care, client (patient) satisfaction, provider participation, rate setting, administrative costs and feasibility, and quality-of-care monitoring and assurance. Although we have alluded to some of these issues throughout, and some are addressed in detail in the component studies themselves, we did not investigate them thoroughly for our integrative study. A simple example would be to ask how the three prototypes differ in their acceptability to Medicaid beneficiaries. The answer to this highly important question remains unknown.

The final limitation that must be acknowledged is that we could have synthesized and presented the accumulated data in our report in a wide variety of ways. The approach and style we selected reflect the perspectives and preferences of the authors. Our chosen approach also allowed us to accommodate disparate program designs and source evaluation studies. We found that every individual study had its own set of acknowledged, and sometimes unacknowledged, limitations. The basic challenge for us was to maximize the use of the accumulated experience while critically appraising the quality of that evidence.

Surmounting Selected Methodological Obstacles

Reviewing and appraising the evaluation evidence permitted us to identify some of the more persistent methodological problems that have plagued the programs' studies. Four important problems and concerns are summarized here.

Person-level files

Perhaps the most problematic issue for evaluators has been the lack of person-specific information that aggregates cost and utilization history for the individual beneficiary. This problem is endemic to research using claims-based data bases, which are primarily designed to process and pay line-item or service-level claims. Moreover, state Medicaid program reporting to the federal government has not required the development of person-level files. State Medicaid agencies only have to report aggregated counts of beneficiaries, the dollars expended, and counts of units of service by broad service categories. None of these requirements necessitates constructing person-specific utilization histories. Few states routinely do so, although some states participate in the Medicaid Tape-to-Tape Project (Baugh, Pine, and Howell 1987), and increasing numbers of states are participating in the HCFA Medicaid Statistical Information System (MSIS) (Cherlow et al. 1991). Both Tape-to-Tape and MSIS produce uniform person-level files. Although lack of resources is a major hindrance for developing person-level data systems, their development would be extremely useful for more focused and detailed monitoring of many aspects of Medicaid operations.

By merging eligibility and utilization data, virtually any state can construct person-level analysis files if they invest the resources, and if providers submit (report) the necessary data, as noted below. However, few states are doing person-level analyses for their program waiver renewal applications. In the absence of this level of detail, program evaluations are greatly handicapped in the methodological and statistical approaches they can use. Some important analyses, such as tests for selection bias, cannot be done at all in the absence of such files. Ten of the 12 studies we selected as "more reliable" used person-level files, although this characteristic was not a specific criterion for inclusion in the subset.

Encounter reporting in capitated programs

The underreporting problem in capitated systems has been a source of controversy and embarrassment for providers, sponsors, and evaluators in several programs. It has been a source of contention and consternation between federal and state officials, and program managers and capitated providers. There have also been serious cost consequences as entire program evaluations have been severely compromised by uncorrectable or uncorrected underreporting.

Critics of reliance on pseudoclaims have suggested they are also called "dummy claims" because only "dummies" would believe them. Others view them as entirely unnecessary since they are an inefficient way to monitor contractual performance (i.e., case by case).

The current unsatisfactory approaches could be replaced with the following strategy. Rather than requiring prepaid plans and providers to report encounters to the Medicaid agency in a manner that is similar to claims, including integrating and processing them in the state Medicaid management information system as "no pay" claims, administrators could limit the reporting requirement to aggregate encounter data only. However, plans would have to demonstrate that their internal management information systems maintain a minimum data set for each service encounter. In addition, these data would have to be retrievable on demand by the state agency or its agents (evaluators) in machine-readable fashion. Thus, evaluators could effectively bypass state-level data systems and deal directly with plans or provider groups. The minimum data set would be designed with a reasonable level of clinical and administrative detail. Given the growing demands on prepaid plans by private sector purchasers, this would not be an unfair burden or unreasonable expectation.

Before and after and comparison group designs

A surprising number of program evaluations have serious flaws in the design of the contrasts intended to isolate and demonstrate program impacts. The use of either naive or heroic assumptions about past trends continuing into the future too often provides a dubious reference point against which to compare observed experience. Likewise, selecting comparison groups that are not comparable, or whose comparability cannot be adequately established, casts doubt on the credibility of what might in truth be a highly successful program. In both instances, the problem is exacerbated by the lack of person-level detail that could support more legitimate modeling and isolation of program effects. The fact that some rather weak designs have sufficed to meet waiver renewal requirements raises questions about the rigor and integrity of the waiver review process. State agencies obviously recognize this problem as well and might conclude that improved evaluation efforts are not necessary.

Evaluating inpatient effects

Nearly 80 percent of the programs we studied here reported reductions in inpatient use, many of which were substantial. Despite the reductions in these high-cost services, the amount of savings reported in these same programs was more modest. Previously, we asked two questions about these savings: Are they credible, and can they be attributed to the gatekeeper intervention? The latter question has already been discussed in detail. We argued earlier that designs that made more serious efforts to clearly link the gatekeeper intervention to program effects tended to find weaker inpatient effects. With respect to the former question of credibility, there is some evidence that a number of the prepaid programs are susceptible to a so-called preenrollment window trap that might understate inpatient use in capitated programs. As described in Chapter 5, newly eligible beneficiaries cannot be instantaneously enrolled with a plan or gatekeeper. Since the newly eligibles typically have high initial use, this use might occur before enrollment and thus be paid for by the conventional Medicaid program. The level of detail available in most of these analyses precludes establishing that this use is or is not occurring. However, some of the larger programs have already identified this problem. Thus, the preenrollment window effect is a lurking problem that future evaluators will need to explicitly rule out.

Priority Issues for Future Primary Care Case Management Research

We conclude our study of the accumulated use and cost impact evidence from the first decade of PCCM by enumerating several research issues that should receive priority consideration.

What are the longitudinal effects of PCCM programs? Studies are needed to identify whether initially observed use and cost effects remain the same, intensify, or evaporate as programs move into maturity and steady state.

Will the apparent savings in Type 1 programs hold up under rigorous evaluation designs? Some of these programs have reported the largest aggregate savings in the PCCM experience by virtue of large enrollment, ease of implementation, and long duration. However, serious questions about the validity of their asserted savings have been raised. As more states look to this appealing strategy, this question requires a definitive response.

Do programs in which states contract with HMOs and HIOs, and thereby obtain guaranteed savings, alter the levels of service use and resources consumed by beneficiaries? Studies are needed to go beyond savings by contract to see whether prepaid entities render care in a discernably different manner. This investigation would not only allow a look at the adequacy of care in these entities but also provide insight into the adequacy of the payment rates that states and their contractors are agreeing to accept.

Do two-tiered Type 2 programs that use an intermediary organization to pool risk and to receive and disburse capitation payments represent a distinct program type? If so, how does their cost and use experience compare with that for the other program types? The use of intermediary organizations to expand participation and share risk is both popular and poorly understood. The need for this type of research is suggested by Hillman, Pauly, and Kerstein (1989).

What are some of the detailed dynamics involved in PCCM, including the extent of substitution of alternative forms of care? The level of detail available in most program evaluations has not permitted us to answer many important questions about how patterns of service delivery may be changing. Given the propensity of many program managers to employ incentive systems to alter provider behavior, there is a critical need to collect and analyze data that can further explore the behavioral dynamics of gatekeeping.

Do physicians who move from being primary care managers to primary care gatekeepers change their service delivery behaviors? It has been suggested that becoming gatekeepers will encourage physicians to refer less frequently. In doing so, one might assume they are expanding the range of services they are rendering or the scope of conditions they choose to treat directly. To assess this hypothesized behavior, it is necessary to examine changes with the physician-gatekeeper as the explicit unit of analysis.

Does primary care gatekeeping change the nature of relationships between PCPs and specialists? If program designs channel beneficiaries to PCPs and restrict access to specialists only via physician-made referrals, do these designs alter the status and stature of PCPs vis-à-vis specialists? These designs are similar to many now commonly found in the private sector, which will further contribute to the potential for interspecialty rivalry and conflict. The introduction of RBRVS is almost certain to further contribute to these relationship changes.

Are primary care gatekeeping effects uniform across all covered populations, such as adults and children, or would these programs benefit from more focused targeting of beneficiaries? Our study has looked only at programs covering the AFDC population, with adult and child experience combined in the majority of programs. There is some evidence there are differential effects for these groups when they are studied separately. More generally, there are many unanswered questions about the potential effectiveness of gatekeeping based on different eligibility groups, and on past patterns of utilization of program enrollees, such as high or low users. These issues should be addressed in light of the expected proliferation of gatekeeper programs across Medicaid.

Do the substantial reductions in emergency department use indicate forgone care or care appropriately diverted to primary care practitioners? Are these reductions due to enrollee or provider behavioral changes, or both? Because emergency department use demonstrates the most pervasive impact of PCCM, more study is needed to explain the causes and consequences of these reductions. Is access being directly or subtly redirected to other sites? Does having a guaranteed "medical home" result in enrollees making more phone calls for assistance or reassurance? Do increases in primary care visits compensate for some or all of these reduced emergency department visits?

Should primary care gatekeeping programs attempt to maximize the participation of existing regular sources of care? A key current debate in managed care initiatives in both public and private sectors concerns the selection of participating providers. However, when a program selects a subset of providers, it excludes others, which can diminish overall participation and thereby access. Does provider selection produce disruption and dislocation in patient-provider relationships? Does selection have a detectable effect on expected program outcomes? A related question is whether providers who have typically participated in Medicaid can be persuaded to do so under new arrangements.

Can the expected benefits of primary care gatekeeping be obtained when enrollees are not formally linked with an identified physician by the organization with which they enrolled? This question is particularly germane to Type 3 programs and can be posed more directly as follows: Can and do organizations perform the gatekeeping function as effectively as do individual physicians?

Conclusion

This study of the structure and selected outcome experience from 25 PCCM programs developed in Medicaid in the past decade provides an important compendium of the current state of knowledge. Although it is neither exhaustive nor definitive in many respects, it should reduce much of the confusion about the PCCM strategy that has accumulated during its first decade. As the 1990s unfold, the issues we examined here will need to be revisited and the evidence updated. There is obviously much more to learn.

References

Baugh, D., P. Pine, and E. Howell. 1987. "The Medicaid Tape-to-Tape Project: A Design for Medicaid Research." Paper prepared for the 25th Annual Meeting of the National Association of Welfare Research and Statistics, Baltimore, MD.

Buchanan, J., A. Leibowitz, J. Keesey, J. Mann, and C. Damberg. 1992. *Cost and Use of Capitated Medical Services: Evaluation of the Program for Prepaid Managed Health Care.* RAND/UCLA/Harvard Center for Health Care Financing Policy Research. Santa Monica, CA: RAND Corporation.

Cherlow, A., M. R. Ellwood, E. Howell, K. Miller, and S. Dodds. 1991. "Data Quality in the Medicaid Statistical Information System (MSIS)." Working paper (December). Lexington, MA: SysteMetrics/McGraw-Hill.

Hillman, A. L., M. V. Pauly, and J. J. Kerstein. 1989. "How Do Financial Incentives Affect Physicians' Clinical Decisions and the Financial Performance of HMOs?" *New England Journal of Medicine* 321(2): 86–92.

Hohlen, M., L. Manheim, G. Fleming, S. Davidson, B. Yudkowsky, S. Wermer, and G. Wheatley. 1990. "Access to Office-Based Physicians Under Capitation Reimbursement and Medicaid Case Management: Findings from the Children's Medicaid Program." *Medical Care* 28(1): 59–68.

Hunter, J., T. Schmidt, and G. Jackson. 1982. *Meta-Analysis: Cumulating Research Findings Across Studies.* Beverly Hills, CA: Sage Publications.

Hurley, R., and D. Freund. 1988. "A Typology of Medicaid Managed Care." *Medical Care* 26(8): 764–73.

Light, R. and D. Pillemer. 1984. *Summing Up: The Science of Revisiting Research.* Cambridge, MA: Harvard University Press.

Appendix: Program Descriptions

Contents

Introduction

The following summaries of 25 individual programs are intended to provide the reader with a general overview of program designs and key operational features. They also summarize the methodology employed in evaluating each program and the relevant findings from each evaluation. Finally, each summary includes an assessment of the general contribution of each evaluation. These summaries are of necessity only a brief recapitulation of the enormous volume of information available on each program. The interested reader is encouraged to obtain and review the more detailed and exhaustive source studies, which are cited in the introductory footnotes. Readers interested in additional or updated information on current Medicaid managed care activities are encouraged to contact

National Academy for State Health Policy
50 Monument Square, Suite 302
Portland, ME 04101
(207) 874-6524

This organization maintains and distributes lists of contact persons in state Medicaid programs and is engaged in gathering and disseminating information nationwide about Medicaid managed care.

Arizona Health Care Cost Containment System

Information sources

The AHCCCS has been the subject of a greater number of studies and publications than any other Medicaid primary care case management program. The definitive source on the program was the HCFA-sponsored, six-year-long evaluation performed by SRI International.* The evaluation examined implementation and operational issues as well as program outcomes including effects on cost, use, access, satisfaction, and quality.

Program description

Before the implementation of AHCCCS in October 1982, Arizona was the only state in the nation without a Medicaid program. Negotiations were undertaken with HCFA to develop a statewide demonstration that would comprise the Arizona Medicaid initiative. Initially, a three-year demonstration waiver was granted; it was

* SRI International, *Evaluation of the Arizona Health Care Cost Containment System: Final Report,* Contract No. HCFA-500-83-0027 (Palo Alto, CA: SRI International, 1989).

later extended, first for four years and then for five additional years (through 1993). The demonstration program incorporated several cost-containment features, including primary care gatekeeping, copayments, freedom-of-choice restrictions, competitive bidding for providers, prepaid financing, and HCFA-to-state capitation payments.

The basic design was to enroll all beneficiaries with PHPs (Type 3). The health plans would qualify for participation based on competitive bids that they would submit to provide services in designated counties. All Medicaid-eligible persons would be required to choose a qualified plan or be assigned to one (with low-bidder providers receiving most auto-assignees). In 1988 the program had approximately 226,000 enrollees, of whom half were AFDC beneficiaries. Over the first six years of the programs, 22 PHPs participated, with enrollments ranging from 500 to 50,000; but by 1988, the number of plans stood at 13.

Plans submitted bids to provide all covered services (long-term care was initially excluded) in targeted counties, and multiple providers were selected to ensure enrollee choice. Plans were paid their bid rate or a negotiated price that resulted from a best-and-final bid. The plans were required to implement primary care gatekeeping and to use nominal copayments as a utilization control feature. Evidence suggests that there was wide variation in the extent of both of these features, as discussed in the findings. Plans could be (1) preexisting HMOs or (2) specifically organized PHPs composed of physician networks or programs sponsored by hospital outpatient clinics.

The SRI report details three distinct phases in the development of AHCCCS—startup (and difficulties), recovery, and stabilization—suggesting that an understanding of program effects needs to be conditioned on recognizing these differing contexts. Serious problems arose with the private contractor administering the program, especially in the information and enrollment realm. These problems ultimately led to contract termination and state assumption of these program duties. One of the consequences of these difficulties was that certain program features such as the management information system (MIS), encounter reporting, and quality assurance, were seriously delayed in their development. Although this has been a common experience in many Medicaid managed-care initiatives, the implications, especially for the evaluation of AHCCCS, were quite serious.

Research method

The scope of SRI's evaluation contract included implementation, operational, and outcome assessments. To accomplish these tasks a variety of data sources and collection techniques were planned, some of which were never implemented (e.g., the physician survey) or were seriously compromised by data quality and availability (cost and use analysis). However, consumer surveys were done to examine satisfaction, access, use, and quality through the use of comparison groups selected from New Mexico's Medicaid program. In addition, multiple estimates of program "savings" were presented.

There are several particularly thorny problems in evaluating AHCCCS. The first of these is that there was no prior Medicaid program, so a before and after design was not possible. Thus, the AHCCCS program design intervention effect could not be disentangled from an insurance intervention effect. Because it was a statewide program, there was no in-state comparison group under conventional Medicaid. This situation required the use of other states for comparative information, which introduced other confounding factors. The AHCCCS program intervention introduced several features concurrently, such as prepayment, gatekeeping and restricted choice, copayments, etc., which prevented attributing observed changes to specific features. Yet another problem was that PHPs do not routinely produce claims data for monitoring utilization. To acquire such data, federal (and ultimately state) authorities attempted to mandate that plans submit pseudoclaims or encounter data. Finally, the basic question of how to estimate savings was necessarily difficult and arbitrary for several of the reasons noted above.

Findings

The asserted program savings for AHCCCS were calculated in two ways and from two perspectives (state and federal), as detailed in the SRI final report. The first way was called prospective and was based on the cost of equivalent Medicaid programs. Federal capitation to the state was initially set at 95 percent of a prospective estimate of the cost of a Medicaid program in Arizona, thus accruing a 5 percent savings by definition. Net savings for AFDC and Supplemental Security Income (SSI) enrollees only were estimated to be $15.3 million over the first five years. The other approach, referred to as retrospective, examined rates of increases in comparison states that had programs similar in coverage to that of Arizona. Aged, disabled, and AFDC groups were separately analyzed. This approach found that Arizona's expenditures increased by an average rate of 10.4 percent over this time, or aggregate savings of $33.8 million. Examining only per capita expenditures for medical services, the annual rate of increase was 5.3 percent in Arizona versus 8.2 percent in the comparison states, or a full 3 percent lower.

Unfortunately, the findings regarding utilization effects were far less clear or authoritative. The analysis did not have either a before and after or a comparison group design with which to perform necessary contrasts. Therefore, the measures of 553 days per 1,000 and 4.3 physician visits for AFDC enrollees are rather uninformative. Moreover, even these data are suspect given the enormous problems, well detailed by SRI, in getting plans to submit usable encounter data. Plan-by-plan analyses underscore the unevenness in compliance and thus raise serious doubts about the credibility of all utilization findings. The only attempt to provide a comparative frame of reference used a highly disparate set of indicators that merely suggested the findings are potentially on target. There was some assessment of the extent of underreporting, such as 10 percent for inpatient stays, that were informative and credible, but again no valid comparison group was employed.

There were comparison groups used in the access and satisfaction and the quality-of-care studies, namely samples from the New Mexico Medicaid programs. Though these were small sample-studies, they cast some light on some utilization impacts. For example, there is an indication that beneficiaries found access to emergency department care more restricted in Arizona than in New Mexico, consistent with the gatekeeping feature of the program. On the other hand, routine care was seen as more accessible in Arizona than in New Mexico when every person was formally enrolled with a responsible plan and gatekeeper.

Assessment

The AHCCCS is such a unique program that its contribution to an understanding of the broader phenomenon of managed care in Medicaid is somewhat limited. Its use of competitive bidding is perhaps its most distinctive feature, but evidence suggests that the extent of competition has steadily declined over the life of the program. With respect to primary care gatekeeping, SRI reported that its use by participating plans was far from universal (strongest in IPAs and HMOs and weakest in clinic-based plans). Apparently the use of copayments was also unevenly implemented and is rather rare in Medicaid managed-care programs, which have frequently eliminated their use when beneficiaries have given up freedom of choice.

With respect to the evaluation, the SRI study has many strengths, especially in terms of implementation, operation, competitive bidding, and quality of care. It is less strong in its analysis of cost impacts, in part because of the unique status of the program. Unfortunately, its weakest part is its assessment of the impact of the program on utilization. These findings are subject to serious underreporting bias.

Monterey County (California) Health Initiative

Information sources

The source for this study was Research Triangle Institute's (RTI's) MCD evaluation and various publications using data accumulated during the evaluation.*

Program description

The Monterey program was established as an HIO that contracted with the Medi-Cal program to enroll all AFDC beneficiaries with PCPs and health care organizations, which would function as primary care managers. Approximately 22,000 persons were eligible. The program was originally intended to pay these providers capitation for primary care with the possibility of shared savings opportunities from reductions in referral care use. Resistance from the medical community ultimately led to redesigning the payment methods to FFS plus a monthly case management fee (Type 1).

Implemented in 1983, the program began to experience financial problems early due to serious administrative difficulties, including a nonfunctioning MIS.

---

* Research Triangle Institute (RTI), *Evaluation of the Medicaid Competition Demonstrations: Integrative Final Report,* HCFA Contract No. 500-83-0050 (Research Triangle Park, NC: Research Triangle Institute, 1989); S. Garfinkel, W. Zelman, F. Bryan, and D. Freund, *Financial Problems Contributing to the Insolvency of the Monterey Health Initiative,* HCFA Contract No. 500-83-0050 (Research Triangle Park, NC: Research Triangle Institute, 1985); B. Aved, "The Monterey County Health Initiative: A Post-Mortem Analysis of a California Demonstration Project," *Medical Care* 25, no. 1 (1987): 35–45.

Moreover, adopting FFS as the payment method without utilization monitoring or control made changes in utilization unlikely. Because the contract with Medi-Cal involved paying the Monterey HIO a capitation rate that was discounted from expected FFS, the utilization reductions would have had to be sufficient to offset both this discount and the administrative costs associated with operating what was essentially a local version of the state Medicaid program. The lack of reductions ultimately led to insolvency despite some last-ditch efforts to salvage the program by changing fees and bolstering utilization review. The program was discontinued in 1985, and Medi-Cal eligibles reverted to customary freedom-of-choice, FFS benefits. The ailing nature of the program in its final year makes data from that period unreliable.

Research method

Since the method of payment remained FFS, the Monterey program presents an opportunity to examine the impact of imposing the gatekeeper role unconfounded by a concomitant change in the method of payment (one large hospital outpatient department was an exception to this arrangement).

The general analytical approach used in the RTI study to assess cost and use effects was a quasi-experimental design with a before and after nonequivalent comparison group. Data were extracted from claims files for stratified random samples of approximately 2,000 children and 1,000 adults for the demonstration county and a comparison county (Ventura) for the year before the demonstration and the first year of the demonstration. Person-level utilization and cost files were built for each person in the samples for developing mean levels of cost and use. Using data from eligibility files for sample members, evaluators developed multivariate models of use for several use measures employing the RAND two-part model of use: probability of use and use levels for users only.

Measures of use were available for inpatient admissions and days, physician visits by specialty, emergency department use, ancillary use, care concentration, and, though not previously reported, prescription use. The analysis of program effects assessed the impact of being in the demonstration site in the demonstration year after controlling for age, gender, duration of eligibility, continuous versus noncontinuous eligibility, the presence of other insurance coverage, site, and year. In other words, the rate of change in use and cost in the demonstration site was compared to the change in the comparison site. Because FFS was the method of payment, there was no risk of underreporting, nor was there a selection bias issue since this program was mandatory. As such, the Monterey analysis is potentially generalizable to other Type 1 PCCM programs.

Findings

The results for use effects are available for adults and children, but the cost effects are consolidated since the capitation rate used between the state and the HIO was a combined one. The only significant effect on inpatient use was a reduction of 17 percent in days per thousand for children; admission rates were unchanged relative to the comparison groups. Emergency department use was markedly lower with reductions in excess of 35 percent for adults and children in the probability of at least one emergency department visit.

Total physician visits declined by 15 percent for children and 2 percent for adults. Detailed analysis indicated that sharp reductions for both groups in specialist contacts were partially offset by increases in PCP visits. Prescription use, which was not analyzed in multivariate models, was lower by approximately 20 percent for children and 10 percent for adults.

The expected FFS per capita payment in the demonstration year was $606 (versus $603 in the year before). The capitation payment made to the HIO was $670, suggesting that the state actually paid more than it would have under FFS. However, because of the capitation rate discount and the administrative costs due to the program—including the case management fee—the HIO actually had approximately 90 percent of the FFS equivalent rate available to pay for medical services. It was the magnitude of this shortfall that ultimately caused the program to be dissolved in bankruptcy, notwithstanding some discernable effects on utilization solely due to gatekeeping without financial risk.

Assessment

This is a complete and useful person-level analysis with large representative samples from a before and after comparison group design. Because the method of payment was not altered, the data source is essentially comparable from year to year and across sites. The evaluation of gatekeeping can be independent of changes or differences in method of payment. Several measures of use were employed, most of which display good stability in the comparison site. The analysis controlled for several potential influences on use and cost, although not for prior use, because the samples were not panels of continuously eligible persons.

The principal weakness of the study lies in its only analyzing the first year of operation, which would have been affected by a variety of factors that would not continue to be important over a sustained period. This is a problem with all the MCD studies, but since Monterey had a relatively short existence, later data either would not have been available or could have been contaminated by the widely observed impending bankruptcy. This latter point must also be recognized as a limitation on the overall contribution of the Monterey evaluation.

Health Plan of San Mateo County (California)

Information sources

The two principal sources for information on this program were the waiver renewal application dated August 1989 and a report on the structural and incentive features of the program contained in "Giving Physicians Incentives to Contain Costs Under

Medicare: Lessons from Medicaid''—an Urban Institute Working Paper by Welch, subsequently published in the *Health Care Financiang Review.**

Program description

The Health Plan of San Mateo (HPSM) is operated as an HIO by a county-based commission that contracts with the state Medi-Cal program. The capitation is based on 95 percent of expected FFS expenditures. The HPSM receives a supplemental payment that represents the state's expected reduction in administrative cost due to subcontracting program responsibilities to the HIO. The plan became operational in December 1987. As a mandatory program it currently is responsible for providing virtually all Medicaid services to eligible residents. At the end of 1990 this group represented approximately 31,000 beneficiaries. The basic program design is a primary care gatekeeping network, and beneficiaries must select and enroll with a primary care manager who provides primary care and authorizes all referral care, including inpatient care.

Primary care managers are at some financial risk in the program (Type 2). They are paid a capitation for primary care services, 20 percent of which is withheld until settlement. In addition, in one of the most novel aspects of this program, physicians are organized around county hospitals for the purpose of pooling risk for referral (specialty) care, inpatient services, and other services including drugs and outpatient care. Each physician must declare his or her principal affiliating hospital. Depending on the performance of both the individual physician and the hospital pool as manifested by balances in the various accounts, year-end settlements are made per a risk-sharing formula among the physician, the hospital, and the HPSM. In essence, the goal is to encourage reduction in referral, hospital, and other use to enable the primary care manager to receive the capitation withholding and perhaps a share of residuals in other accounts. The HIO determines how the specialists, hospital, and other providers are paid, with the hospitals sharing in the risk arrangement.

As with the Santa Barbara program described below, one of the goals of the HPSM is to enable local authorities and providers to develop a decentralized, and potentially more customized, Medicaid program. It is believed that fashioning an alternative delivery system in this manner will improve participation, enhance administration-provider communication, and promote a high-quality delivery system.

Research method

The HPSM has not yet been extensively evaluated since it has been under way only since 1988. The only currently available sources for information are the brief cost-effectiveness assessment in the 1989 waiver renewal application, limited data reported by Welch, and communication with the executive director of the HPSM

* W. P. Welch, ''Giving Physicians Incentives to Contain Costs Under Medicaid,'' *Health Care Financing Review* 12, no. 2 (1990): 103–12.

regarding inpatient experience. Given issues regarding claims runout time, the availability of comparison groups, and other logistical issues in analyzing claims data, it is not clear when more definitive data will be forthcoming. Thus, the limited findings available are reported below with necessary caveats.

Findings

The structural arrangements between Medi-Cal and the HIO guarantee some up-front savings per the contract that pays a capitation rate of 95 percent of the expected FFS rate for each enrollee (rates vary by age, gender, and eligibility category). However, the state also pays a supplement fee that represents reduced state operating expenses, given that the HPSM assumed most Medi-Cal responsibilities. The supplement fee thereby reduces the state's overall expected savings. Based on the computations state officials did in the waiver application, the program resulted in savings of approximately $700,000, or 3 percent, during the first seven months of 1988.

The executive director suggested that the savings observed were probably caused by reductions in inpatient use. In December 1990, hospital days per thousand were estimated to be between 975 and 985 for all eligible groups, which was approximately 100 days (or 10 percent) lower than historical experience. This reduction was attributed to both case management and other utilization review activities employed by the HPSM. Welch's information, based on the 1988 experience of the five-hospital risk pool, suggested that "overall, physicians are breaking even."* Payments to hospitals were very close to their per diems, again suggesting that modest reductions in use resulted in payments that approached expected rates. Unfortunately, there are no data on physician services other than that physician payments also approached expected rates, perhaps indicating minimal changes in service volume. It is also important to note that since primary care services are capitated, the unavailability of encounter data is certain to be problematic.

Assessment

The limited operational experience in San Mateo provides us with limited evidence at this point. However, the creative use of hospital-based risk pools merits close study in the future to ascertain whether this is a viable vehicle for constructing and sustaining a primary care network with substantial risk sharing. In particular, comparative analyses of Santa Barbara and San Mateo will be informative from a structural standpoint since they represent alternative approaches to Type 2 PCCM.

---

* Welch, "Giving Physicians Incentives," 111.

Santa Barbara County (California) Health Initiative

Information sources

The study sources were RTI's MCDs evaluation* and various publications using data accumulated during the evaluation.

Program description

The Santa Barbara program was established as an HIO in 1983 and continues to the present time as the Medi-Cal program in the county. As an HIO it annually negotiates a capitated rate with the state to provide virtually all Medi-Cal services to all Medi-Cal beneficiaries in the county, who number about 25,000. The basic program design is to make capitated payments to PCPs for the primary care services of beneficiaries who are enrolled. These primary care managers are also able to participate in shared savings in the residuals in referral accounts, making this a Type 2 model program. A substantial portion of the eligible populations (estimated at 20 percent) is enrolled with capitated county health clinics, which also function as primary care managers with salaried staff physicians.

The program has witnessed a substantial amount of conflict between the state and the HIO over rates, which the HIO has persistently argued have been insufficient and inappropriate, according to its calculations. The program also experienced some initial problems in developing MIS capacity, including the ability to provide timely, reliable information on enrollment and utilization. These problems ultimately were resolved, although their effects might have influenced early operating experience.

Research method

This program introduced both primary care gatekeeping and capitation for primary care services with shared savings opportunities. As such, the analyses performed were unable to disentangle these two components.

The general analytical approach used in the RTI study to assess cost and use effects was a quasi-experimental design with a before and after nonequivalent comparison group. Data were extracted for claims for stratified random samples of approximately 2,000 children and 1,000 adults for the demonstration county and a comparison county (Ventura County) for the year before the demonstration and the first year of the demonstration. Person-level utilization cost files were built for each person in the samples for use in developing mean levels of cost and use. Using data from eligibility files for sample members, researchers developed multivariate models of use for several use measures employing the RAND two-part model of use: probability of use and use for users only.

---

* Research Triangle Institute (RTI), *Evaluation of the Medicaid Competition Demonstrations: Integrative Final Report,* HCFA Contract No. 500-83-0050 (Research Triangle Park, NC: Research Triangle Institute, 1989).

Measures of use were available for inpatient admissions and days, physician visits by specialty, emergency department use, ancillary use, care concentration, and, though not previously reported, prescription use. The analysis of program effects assessed the impact of being the demonstration site in the demonstration year after controlling for a number of person-level variables. A potential problem, given the capitation payment for primary care services, was underreporting of encounters. Providers were required to submit pseudoclaims for these services, but detailed analysis suggests that underreporting did occur and was most pronounced for enrollees in county health clinics. As it was a mandatory program, selection bias affecting the analysis was not a problem.

In addition to this cost and use analysis with claims data, the Santa Barbara program was also analyzed via a Medicaid consumer survey with both AFDC and SSI beneficiaries and a quality-of-care study, both of which employed Ventura County as the comparison site. While highly informative on a number of program features, the findings from the claims data analysis are viewed as the most definitive with respect to cost and use effects.

Findings

The results of the analyses are available for adults and children in terms of use effects but are combined for cost effects because the capitation payment to the HIO was consolidated in California. The only significant decrease in inpatient use was found for the probability that a child would be admitted (a decrease of 32 percent). Emergency department use was 28 percent lower for children and 30 percent lower for adults. Physician services use was lower by about 20 percent. Part of the reduction was due to substantial reductions in specialist contacts, although PCP visits also were lower (in part because of the shifting of care to county health clinics away from physician offices). The underreporting of primary care services also led to lower levels of use. Prescription use was also lower for children (by approximately 25 percent) and for adults (15 percent).

The cost findings for Santa Barbara indicate that actual expenditures by the state were less than projected using the FFS expectation ($677 versus $708), although this reduction was not statistically significant. This did represent about a 10 percent reduction from the prior year, suggesting that the program did achieve some cost containment, particularly given the 20 percent increase observed in the comparison county. Adding back administrative costs increased per capita expenditures to a point close to, if not in excess of, capitation payments. Because of this, the program has been under cash constraints for much of its existence. This situation has added pressure to the annual negotiations with the state to ensure adequate capitation rates paid on a timely basis.

No detailed cost and use analysis has been performed since the MCD studies, which applied only to the developmental years of the program.

Assessment

Like all the MCD studies, this analysis is generally well done with large samples from claims data in the context of a good research design. However, the underreporting issue is a problem in Santa Barbara, whereas it was not in Monterey, for example. Moreover, contemporaneous changes in gatekeeping and method of payment make it impossible to attribute findings to either of these program features. The use of a comparison site enables some control for history effects, but the effects of program maturation are unexplored here. This program has now been in operation for four years since the detailed analysis was conducted.

Despite the time-bound nature of the Santa Barbara study, the results are well triangulated by the availability of consumer survey findings and a quality-of-care study. Both of these provide one the most comprehensive, wholistic pictures of a primary care case management program in Medicaid. Inasmuch as the effects and lack of effects are corroborated across these three sources, a high level of confidence in the findings, at least regarding the early days of the Santa Barbara program, is justified.

Colorado Primary Care Physician Program

Information sources

The study sources were an evaluation report prepared by the University of Colorado Health Sciences Center* and the 1989 waiver renewal application by the state. Additional background information was available from the MPE 1988 report.†

Program description

The Primary Care Physician Program (PCPP) is a mandatory enrollment program for all Medicaid beneficiaries except those in foster care, those dually certified, and those with SSI benefits. Those beneficiaries who choose to enroll voluntarily in an HMO are exempted from the PCPP mandate. The program was initiated in 1982 and had approximately 72,000 enrollees in 1988. The program experienced some problems in achieving full coverage but now has sufficient PCP capacity in all but 5 of the state's 63 counties.

Beneficiaries enroll with their PCP of choice. That physician agrees to provide, broker, or authorize virtually all care except emergencies, including early and periodic screening, diagnosis, and treatment (EPSDT); family planning services; and dental services. Primary care physicians are paid FFS (Type 1). Initially, they were also provided with annual incentive payments, but these appear to have been discontinued now per the most recent evaluation. There appears to be a high level of physician acceptance of the program, and the mean number of enrollees is 35 per participating physician.

* G. E. Fryer, "Evaluation of the Primary Care Physician Program" (Denver, CO: Health Sciences Center, University of Colorado, 1986 and 1988).

† Office of Research and Demonstrations (ORD), *Medicaid Program Evaluation: Final Report*, Report No. MPE 9.2, eds. J. Holahan, J. Bell, and G. S. Adler (Baltimore, MD: Health Care Financing Administration, 1987).

Research method

Similar program evaluations were conducted in 1986 and 1988 by the University of Colorado. The approach used was to examine the experience of a representative sample of 2,000 persons who had completed their first year in the PCPP and compare it to the utilization and cost experience in conventional Medicaid in the year before enrollment. This approach meant the population being examined had to have two years of continuous eligibility. The focus of the analysis was the impact of gatekeeping since the method of payment had not been altered.

The approach was described by the analyst as a one-group, before and after design, which in effect used the group as its own control. No comparison group was employed. Age- and gender-adjusted rates of use were presented to better probe the data and to examine its comparability to other data bases. The data sources were claims as well as a brief consumer attitude survey mailed to approximately 1,700 new beneficiaries with a response rate of nearly 50 percent. The measures available for use and cost analysis included inpatient admissions and expenditures, physician visits and expenditures, outpatient clinic visits and expenditures (which included emergency department visits), and total expenditures, all of which were presented per person. Statistical tests were conducted on the rates for the years before and after implementation. Selection bias impact on effects due to voluntary enrollees opting out of PCPP was not discussed.

Findings

The 1988 evaluation reported a reduction in admissions from 181 per 1,000 to 116 per 1,000. A statistically significant savings of 26 percent in inpatient expenditures per person was realized. The analysis then applied this savings of $129 per beneficiary to the entire enrolled population of 72,000 to arrive at an estimated inpatient savings of $9.3 million. Outpatient savings were more modest, although the average number of outpatient visits per person declined by a statistically significant amount from 2.0 to 1.87. Estimated savings reached $322,000. Physician visits increased from 4.7 to 5.6 visits per person per year, and expenditures for these services increased by approximately $91 per year. Both changes were statistically significant. The analysis suggests this increase in physician visits represented a substitution of such services for both inpatient and outpatient services.

The overall cost effectiveness of the program was the net of service expenditures per person and administrative costs, which were less than $2 per beneficiary per year. Overall savings were $3.1 million or $43.45 per beneficiary. The administrative costs included personnel, supplies, and hotline costs, but no claims-processing allocation.

The age and gender adjusted analysis is informative in that it demonstrates that the principal impact of the intervention was on women aged 18 to 44, while the impact on children was limited, and costs actually were higher for the 45- to 65-year-old population. The analyst attributed this impact to the program's influence on the receipt of obstetrical care but did not provide any additional detail on this assertion.

Assessment

The one-group, before and after test design had the advantage of a panel design in that it could examine how use changed in contiguous periods. The measures of cost and use, though limited in number and detail, were subjected to tests of statistical significance. In addition, the age adjustment done here is informative with respect to the potential merits of targeting PCP programs, rather than incorporating all groups and expecting uniform savings. It should be noted, however, that the sampling strategy might have forced newly eligible pregnant women into the year before implementation group, thereby almost ensuring that first year use would be lower.

There are several important limitations with the design and the extrapolation done to calculate statewide savings. The absence of a comparison group makes it impossible to rule out other changes that might have accounted for reductions after enrollment. The inclusion of only continuously eligible persons in the program is also problematic, because of both its nonrepresentativeness of the Medicaid population and the coverage effect associated with new Medicaid eligibility. That is, individuals who are newly eligible might consume more resources in their initial period of eligibility and reach a stable state in use beyond this period; such a finding would be compatible with the reductions reported here. An additional limitation is the lack of data on emergency department use since reductions in outpatient clinic use might occur simply because of site-shifting of outpatient routine care to PCP offices.

The calculation of overall savings by multiplying the rate of savings in the study sample times the total enrolled population is highly questionable. Most fundamentally, this procedure presumed that savings found in the sample group would be obtainable or sustainable for all populations for each year of their enrollment. The analysis done here does not support such an assertion.

In conclusion, the study is informative in several important ways for the sample examined, but its generalizability to the enrolled population as a whole is limited. It is also useful in its attempt to zero in on what population (age and gender) groups are the most amenable to behavior change, assuming these changes are not simply an artifact of the sampling design.

Kansas Primary Care Network

Information sources

The study sources were an internal analysis prepared for the third waiver renewal application and the 1987 MPE study.*

---

* Kansas Department of Social and Rehabilitation Services, "The Primary Care Network Program Evaluation" (Topeka, KS: Office of Planning and Research, 1990); Office of Research and Demonstrations (ORD), *Medicaid Program Evaluation: Final Report*, Report No. MPE 9.2, eds. J. Holahan, J. Bell, and G. S. Adler (Baltimore, MD: Health Care Financing Administration, 1987).

Program description

The Kansas Primary Care Network (PCN) program was initiated in 1984 and currently operates in seven of the most urban counties in the state, with a total enrollment of 78,000 beneficiaries in all noninstitutionalized Medicaid-eligible groups (except for dually eligibles). The program is mandatory in the counties in which it is offered. Beneficiaries must enroll with a PCP or a clinic. The physician or clinic is paid FFS plus a $3 per month fee to provide, broker, and authorize all services to enrollees (Type 1).

The offering of the program only in urban areas is the result of early experience in one rural county indicating that where choice of PCPs is limited by supply factors, little opportunity exists to achieve substantial savings based on choice. Fee-for-service was used because of little statewide experience with HMOs and prepayment and therefore strong resistance to capitation.

Research method

The program covers the above-mentioned eligible groups. Its focal intervention is on the physician as gatekeeper inasmuch as method of payment has not been changed, except for the case management fee. The sources for the analysis were the internal studies conducted by the Kansas Department of Social and Rehabilitation Services for the waiver applications. This was also the source on which the earlier MPE study relied as well.

The evaluators employed trend analysis with comparison and intervention groups. The intervention group comprised the 7 counties in which PCN is offered, and the comparison group comprised the remaining 98 counties in the state without the program. The county experience was the level of analysis, although units of measurement were at the procedural level, as described below. The basic approach was to calculate preimplementation measures of the use of services per eligible in each group. The trended rates of utilization for the comparison counties were then applied to the intervention counties to represent the expected level of use in the intervention counties, that is, had the PCN program not been implemented. The actual rates of use experienced in the PCN counties were computed from claims-paid experience in this FFS program. The savings attributed to the program were the differences between actual and expected levels of use. The cost savings were the use levels times the prices being paid for those services.

Measures of use available in the data were inpatient days, outpatient services (emergency department visits were not separately counted), physician services, and pharmacy services. The outpatient and physician services actually were procedure counts, while pharmacy services were number of prescriptions. The data were reported county by county, and savings were reported for each type of service as well as in aggregate, net of administrative costs and case management fees. Because enrollment was mandatory, there was no threat of selection bias, nor was underreporting of use a problem given FFS payment. A significant problem with the analysis lies in the lack of comparability between the PCN counties, which were distinctly urban, and the counties in the comparison group, which were mostly rural. In addition, the design had the effect of attributing all change in use between expected and actual to the PCN intervention. The fluctuations from year to year suggest that lags in the payment of claims might have contributed to some of the unevenness, although this possibility was not discussed in the analysis.

Findings

In the four-year interval from 1987 through 1990, the net savings reported were $1.2 million, $4.6 million, $0.25 million loss, and $4.7 million, for a total of approximately $10.0 million. Throughout the period, the inpatient savings were the determining factor in the amount of aggregate savings, while physician services in fact increased over expected levels in each of the four years. For 1990, inpatient use was lower than expected, as were outpatient services and prescription services. Inpatient use was about 70 days per 1,000 below a generally expected level of 13 per 1,000 days while outpatient services were 2.36 versus 4.44 procedures per person and prescriptions were 7.95 versus 8.35 prescriptions per person. On the other hand, actual physician procedures were 17.72 versus the expected level of 16.73, which was the smallest difference (loss) yet experienced in this service category.

The state believes that the increase in physician services was to be expected given the program design, as it encouraged both substitution of primary care services and site shifting of care, especially from the outpatient clinic to the physician's office. A related point is based on a consumer survey, in which 49 percent of beneficiaries reported not having a regular physician before enrolling in the PCN. This finding would suggest that physician use might have increased because of the establishment of a contractually obligated available source of care. Only 39 percent of enrollees reported that their PCN physician was their prior regular source of care.

The analysis permits the examination of program effects by individual PCN counties and suggests that the three largest counties were the source of virtually all the savings. This finding is consistent with the state's view that the program effect is directly proportional to the availability of multiple (and thus inefficient) sources of care. Because emergency department use cannot be separated from outpatient use, the likely reduction of emergency department use in urban areas cannot be documented here.

Assessment

The Kansas PCN program is a large, low-intensity intervention on which a number of other states, including Kentucky (and to a lesser extent North Carolina), have modeled their interventions. The availability of four years of county-level information with unit-of-service details is useful. It is especially supportive of the view that the program effect is mediated by local market conditions such as provider availability effects.

The weaknesses of the study lie in the noncomparability of the comparison group of rural counties, the lack of individual-level detail, unexplained substantial fluctuations from year to year in rates of use, and the inability to control for personal characteristic differences given the level of analysis employed. The most fundamental problem is that the design in effect assumes a constant relationship in relative levels of use between the rural and urban counties over six years, and it attributes all differences observed between actual and expected (trended) use rates to the PCN intervention. It completely ignores any other history effects that would confound this attribution. It is because of this particular problem that the overall contribution of this analysis must be considered very limited.

Kentucky Patient Access and Care System

Information sources

The study sources were Kentucky's second waiver renewal request along with the University of Kentucky's KenPAC Program Evaluation of October 1989,* and an unpublished analysis by Miller and Gengler.†

Program description

The KenPAC system, the largest HCFA-approved Medicaid case management system in the United States, was implemented in 1986, enrolling 195,000 AFDC and AFDC-related recipients statewide. Eleven counties were not included in the program due to insufficient numbers of physicians or clinics. There were 1,052 physicians participating in 1986, resulting in a physician-to-enrollee ratio of 1 to 186.

KenPAC falls under the Type 1 classification of Medicaid PCCM programs. It has mandatory enrollment. The state contracts with primary care providers, either PCPs or primary care organizations, to serve as case managers. The case manager is responsible for providing primary care and arranging virtually all other services. Case managers receive FFS payment and an additional $3 per month case-management fee per beneficiary. Other providers are reimbursed on an FFS basis.

Feedback reports are given to all case managers regarding overall utilization patterns. Monthly reports are given to all providers so they can compare themselves to other physicians in terms of their beneficiary panel's utilization rates. Physicians whose panels of beneficiaries deviate more than two standard deviations above statewide utilization rates on any variable are identified and given detailed information regarding services received by each KenPAC enrollee that affect this variable.

In addition to PCPs, clinics and group practices may serve as case managers, but they must meet two criteria: (1) have at least one full-time equivalent physician who falls under program criteria as a PCP and (2) have a common medical record. However, rural health clinics are excepted from the PCP restriction since it is recognized that services in these clinics are often provided by family nurse practitioners.

---

* Independent study conducted by the University of Kentucky School of Public Administration, Lexington, KY. Philip Roeder, Ph.D., Principal Investigator.

† M. Miller and D. Gengler, "Kentucky Patient Access and Care System" (Washington, DC: Urban Institute, 1990).

Enrollees are required to select their own case manager but are randomly assigned to a case manager if they fail to choose their own. Random assignment is done regionally and geographically with regard to age and gender appropriateness.

Several confounding issues in the analysis of the program should be noted. First, mental health, obstetrical, and true emergency department services are excluded from the program. Obstetrics is not viewed as a managed care service. In addition, other Kentucky Medicaid program provisions such as limits on preoperative days, weekend admissions, and procedures provided in the ambulatory setting; optional inpatient procedures; and a limit of 14 inpatient days per episode of illness, might affect the evaluation of the KenPAC program.

Results from the second waiver renewal application

Research methods. The research design employed in the waiver renewal application was a time-series trend analysis. The Winters exponential smoothing forecasting technique was employed in this analysis to obtain forecasted units of service that would have been provided without the implementation of KenPAC. Expected versus actual utilization was compared by type of service. The difference between the actual utilization and the expected utilization without the KenPAC program was attributed to the KenPAC program. The decreased costs associated with the decrease in utilization were viewed as savings. An inflation factor was built into the calculation of projected unit costs to yield expected costs when multiplied by the projected expected units of service.

Service units were procedures. Utilization rates for the following services were measured: independent laboratory procedures, inpatient days, outpatient procedures, physician visits, prescription drugs, etc.

Cost differences (savings) were calculated as expected service units times inflated cost per unit, as compared with actual costs.

There does not appear to have been a problem with underreporting of service use since all services were reimbursed on an FFS basis. However, the trend analysis used in this research attributed all changes in costs and utilization to the intervention. Although selection bias is not a threat here, since the program is mandatory and nearly statewide in scope, it should be noted that there might have been differences between those who selected their PCP themselves and those who were assigned.

Findings. Decreases in inpatient visits, outpatient visits, physician services, and other service units were reported. However, the statistical significance of these decreases was not tested.

Decreases in the costs associated with all the above utilization measures was reported. Again, the statistical significance of the decrease was not tested.

Assessment. Because KenPAC is statewide in scope and one of the most uniform state programs in terms of application, it is generalizable to statewide programs in terms of full savings effects.

However, the primary weakness of analysis lies in that it attributed all cost containment efforts to KenPAC, ignoring the effect of history in terms of other requirements of the state Medicaid program—such as utilization review—that might also have affected utilization and thus cost. In addition, the statistical significance of the reported decreases was not tested due to the type of statistical analysis used.

Results from the University of Kentucky's evaluation

Research method. A multiple interrupted time series (MITS) design was employed. Twenty months of preprogram data, six months of enrollment data, and thirty-four months of postenrollment data were used in the analysis. This analysis compared the preprogram period with postenrollment data to eliminate confounding factors during the enrollment period.

The utilization measures of interest in this analysis were physician visits, laboratory procedures, inpatient days, outpatient visits, and prescription drug use. If laboratory procedures were performed in independent labs, then they were counted under the laboratory variable. If they were performed in the outpatient setting, then they were counted as an outpatient visit.

The single outpatient visits measure included both routine outpatient visits and emergency department use. Unit of services per total eligibles was the unit of analysis. Regression analysis was performed. Covariates of time, program, and season were examined in the analysis.

Findings. Although the direction of the coefficients indicated a decrease in utilization for all the variables, only the decreases detected for laboratory procedures (in independent labs) and outpatient visits were statistically significant.

Since the data used in this analysis did not separate routine outpatient visits from emergency department visits, a separate analysis was performed using 27 months of service claims data. The results of this analysis indicate that there was a reduction in both services.

Assessment. The MITS design offers a better picture of aggregate savings. It had the advantage of allowing the confounding effects due to enrollment to be eliminated from the analysis. The econometric models employed in the statistical analysis allowed the use of tests of significance to ascertain the statistical significance of the decreases associated with the negative coefficients. This offered an advantage over the simple examination of a trend line.

Again, as above, the analysis was limited by attributing all cost containment to the intervention. In addition, procedure, rather than person, was used as the unit of measure. Finally, no cost variables were analyzed.

Louisville (Kentucky) Citicare Program

Information sources

The source of the data with which the Citicare program was assessed was a state-sponsored study by the University of Louisville from which a *Medical Care* article was published by Bonham, Barber, and Gerald.*

Program description

In response to fiscal crises in 1982 at the state and city level in Louisville, Kentucky, state and local officials developed a primary care network program that was operated by an HIO. This HIO was managed by Health America, Inc., an HMO management firm. The program was designed to enroll all AFDC beneficiaries—approximately 40,000 in Jefferson County, which includes Louisville—with participating PCPs, clinics, and health centers. The providers would function as primary care managers directly providing or authorizing virtually all covered services.

The primary care managers were compensated with a capitation payment for all ambulatory care services (Type 2). Each month, the provider received 50 percent of the capitation with 30 percent withheld to meet nonhospital referral care and 20 percent withheld for hospital care. The hospital withholding was designed to meet shortfalls in inpatient accounts that were established for enrollees. If referral care or inpatient care fell below expected levels, providers were paid the residuals in the withholding accounts. Providers were to be at risk for up to 5 percent of the overage in these accounts, but this risk was waived in the first year of participation to promote recruitment. The capitation rates were set based on a 5 percent discount from expected FFS payments, thereby guaranteeing savings to the state. The HIO administrator also received a 2 percent capitation rate fee, thereby leaving approximately 93 percent of funds from which administrative and medical services expenses were to be met.

The program proved operationally feasible for the most part but ultimately was terminated because of provider and, to a lesser extent, client opposition. Part of this opposition from providers was due to resistance to capitation, which resulted in lower participation levels among physicians and proportionately higher participation levels in clinics and health centers. This shift had the effect of forcing substantial disruptions in patient-provider relationships.

Research method

Two household consumer surveys with stratified random samples of Medicaid beneficiaries were conducted by a research team from the University of Louisville in 1983 and 1984, during the year before and first year of the Citicare program. The

* G. Bonham, S. Barber, and M. Gerald, "Use of Health Care Before and During Citicare." *Medical Care* 25, no. 2 (1987): 111–19. *See also* D. A. Freund, *Medicaid Reform: Four Studies of Case Management* (Washington, DC: American Enterprise Institute, 1984).

samples had between 300 and 350 heads of household who responded for themselves and for their children. The survey covered a broad range of issues including background, health status, attitudes, health practices, and utilization for a three-month recall period. In the second survey, a substantial proportion of those interviewed were continuously eligible individuals also interviewed in the earlier survey. The methods to deal with potential nonrandomness in the samples were rough but probably sufficient. Because the samples were random, bivariate analyses alone were presented; significant differences in personal characteristics apparently were not detected.

The measures used to examine use included inpatient admissions—which were hypothesized not to change, ambulatory visits in total and by site, and prescriptions. Ambulatory visits by site focused on whether emergency department use declined as expected and whether site shifting occurred from physician offices to clinics, which participated more willingly as primary care managers. The analysis presented both (1) percent with types of care and (2) care per 1,000 and use rate for the three-month recall period. Additional issues addressed included reasons for emergency department visits and the content of physician visits. Findings on perceived quality of care were also presented.

Findings

The Bonham, Barber, and Gerald study does not address actual resources consumed by beneficiaries in FFS equivalents but does note that the state experienced a 5 percent savings due to its discount on the capitation rate paid by the state to the HIO. Based on utilization findings noted below, one might infer that there were minor reductions in actual resources consumed mainly due to reductions in emergency department use.

With respect to inpatient use, there was no significant effect during Citicare. This is not surprising given the short period and the fact that, as the authors note, the preponderance of inpatient use for AFDC adults was for childbirth. There was a reduction in emergency department use of approximately 40 percent, consistent with program objectives and hypothesized effects. Further evidence presented suggests that this reduction was due to non-health-threatening care reductions, although the results were not statistically significant. Overall ambulatory visits were very slightly lower, which was the result of the reduction in emergency department use, a sharp reduction (more than 20 percent) in doctors' office visits, and a 30 percent increase in health center/clinic visits. This result confirms the expectation that substantial site-shifting occurred.

Regarding the content of visits, there was evidence that laboratory and x-ray services were less likely to be provided in an ambulatory visit, consistent with the incentives in the capitation payment. There also was a lower probability of seeing a physician during an ambulatory visit, perhaps again reflecting the reliance on institutional providers rather than on doctors' offices. There was a significant decrease (18 percent) in the proportion of persons in the second-year sample who had a prescription. Finally, and notably, this study also discovered that there was a significant *increase* in out-of-pocket expenditures for beneficiaries in the Citicare program. The authors do not provide an explanation for this finding, but one possibility might be that the restriction on freedom of choice might have led some individuals to seek and pay for "out-of-plan" (non-Medicaid) services.

Assessment

This study effectively used the results of a well-designed consumer household survey to examine the effects and dynamics of the Citicare program on beneficiary utilization. The small size might have diminished the sensitivity necessary to pick up some findings as significant, but the detailed level of information available compensated for some of this.

Its principal contribution lies in the picture of the effects the PCCM intervention had on patterns of ambulatory use. The large reductions in emergency department use were substantiated by evidence suggesting that "unnecessary use" was being reduced. The ambulatory visit findings illustrate that site shifting due to program design and provider participation did in fact occur, with probably negative implications for continuity and certainly for physician satisfaction. The data on the content of visits also are instructive, suggesting that primary care managers recognized the incentives inherent in the payment system and responded accordingly.

The limitations here, well beyond the researchers' control, include that this evaluation was done early in the program development life cycle and that the program was terminated before full-scale effects might have been noted. Of importance is the fact that the obvious disruption in existing doctor-patient relationships probably had at least an initial impact on patterns of use. For example, 40 percent of enrollees had to be assigned to participating plans because they failed to exercise a choice. Once new relationships were established and stabilized to the primary care manager, levels of utilization might have changed, either up or down.

Michigan Medicaid Capitated Clinic Plan

Information sources

The principal source document for this program was a September 1990 evaluation conducted by Health Management Associates (HMA), as contracted by the Michigan Department of Social Services for inclusion with a waiver renewal application.*

Program description

Michigan offers three alternatives to FFS, freedom-of-choice Medicaid participation that correspond to the three prototypes. Enrollment in HMOs (Type 3) is volun-

* Health Management Associates, Gini Associates, and Michigan Peer Review Organization, "An Evaluation of Cost-Effectiveness, Access to Care and Quality of Care of the Capitated Clinic Plan of the Michigan Medicaid Program" (prepared under contract to the Michigan Department of Social Services, Medical Services Administration, Lansing, MI, 1990).

tary and has been under way since 1971 with an enrollment of approximately 110,000 in 1989. A small number of beneficiaries are voluntarily enrolled in the Clinic Plan (CP) program, which consists of health clinics capitated for nearly all services except inpatient care (Type 2). This is described in a separate summary. The third program is the Physician Sponsor Plan (PSP), which originated in 1982 in Wayne County (Detroit). The program initially was designed to be mandatory with beneficiaries permitted to opt out only if they enrolled with an HMO or in the CP program.

Five ambulatory clinics (initially three) now participate in the CP program, which began in 1983. Beneficiaries may voluntarily enroll with the clinic, which assumes responsibility for managing their care. In return, the clinics are paid a capitated rate for all care except inpatient services. This rate is based on the rate paid to HMOs participating in Michigan's voluntary program with the inpatient component. Clinics may also participate in savings resulting from reductions in nonobstetric inpatient use that exceed 20 percent based on an expected level of use computed from an FFS comparison group. A savings bonus also exists for obstetrics-related stays that is based on average cost of the stay only, since the clinics are not expected to be able to influence the rate of pregnancy among enrollees. The enrollment in the CP program was approximately 9,000 in 1988 and apparently can be initiated by the clinics as well as by the normal social service systems. It is not clear whether the clinics must assign individuals to a specific clinic physician who acts as gatekeeper/case manager.

Research method

The waiver assessment evaluation contains information on access, quality, and provider participation in addition to cost and use assessments, which are the focus of this summary. To study cost effects, expected expenditures for CP enrollees were calculated based on a comparable group of FFS beneficiaries from similar geographic areas. The expenses then were compared to the expenditures for ambulatory care (via the capitation payment) and inpatient care (via regular FFS Medicaid). Separate calculations were made for medical costs, nonobstetric hospitalizations, and mental health hospitalization costs. Administrative adjustments were made.

Utilization was studied by examining a cross-section of the data from an FFS comparison group and data from CP enrollees. Inpatient data were available on all enrollees, but ambulatory data from the capitated clinics were not uniformly available. To compensate for this problem, researchers selected enrollees from three clinics that had encounter data in computer-readable form to study ambulatory utilization effects—specifically, physician visits and laboratory visits. The extent of comparability of these data sources was noted as a potential problem by the evaluators.

Because the program was voluntary, the selection bias issue merited special attention and was addressed by examining levels of prior use. For this purpose, samples of persons with eligibility and FFS participation in 1987 (of whom half subsequently entered the CP) were selected from the years before and after implementation and compared to ascertain whether substantial differences were evident in terms of both use and cost. The analysis also created categories of low, medium, and high users to determine whether these categories had comparable representation in the CP and FFS groups.

One additional approach to investigate access effects was used that merits mention. Use levels by CP enrollees were compared to those for HMO enrollees, PSP enrollees, and the residual FFS population in the state.

Findings

The initial finding of note was that there was evidence found in the analysis of unfavorable selection bias for the plans. Enrollees had higher admission rates for both obstetric and nonobstetric stays than did the comparison group in the year prior to their enrollment, although LOS was shorter. Physician office visits were 20 percent higher, lab tests 50 percent higher, and prescriptions 12 percent higher. Total costs were 13 percent higher with most of this difference attributable to higher inpatient expenditures. In three of the five measures of use, CP enrollees were overrepresented in the high user category in the year prior to enrollment.

With respect to utilization effects (uncorrected for the bias noted above), obstetric inpatient use was lower (90 per 1,000 versus 194 per 1,000), nonobstetric days were lower (310 versus 548 per 1,000), and mental health days were 102 versus 322 per 1,000. In all, this represented a difference of 503 days versus 1,066 or about half as many days despite the higher level in the prior year. Alternately, physician visits in the CP plans were 5.4 versus 3.5 in FFS and lab procedures were 4.9 versus 4.0. These higher levels are notable in that the CP levels came from encounter reports that were susceptible to underreporting.

The overall estimate of net savings was reported to be 15.2 percent as compared to expected expenditures under FFS. The bulk of the savings came from nonobstetric, non-mental-health inpatient expenditures (60 percent of total savings) although the mental health inpatient savings were the largest when calculated as the percentage of expenditures in that service area.

The crude (unadjusted for personal differences) analysis of access found that CP enrollees had the highest level of physician visits (5.3) and the lowest levels of both obstetric and nonobstetric admissions when compared with HMO, PSP, and regular FFS enrollees. Because of noncomparability of populations and data sources, this finding cannot be taken too literally.

Assessment

Even though the CP is a relatively small Type 2 program in Michigan, which has larger Type 1 and 3 programs, the analysis performed is informative in many respects. Perhaps most significantly, this model represents a potentially useful urban adaptation for the PCCM approach, where institutional providers are more common than individual physicians but preexisting HMOs are not in operation. The reported effects on use suggest that the clinics could be doing well financially given the program design and payment methods. In addition, the state's savings clearly have been more substantial than noted in the Michigan PSP.

The evaluators did directly explore evidence of prior use differences but unfortunately did not incorporate this evidence of bias into the analysis of program effects. Thus, one is left with having to infer that the reductions were achieved despite higher prior propensities to use. An alternative explanation could be that prior-year use (postnatal enrollment, for example) could stabilize or decline and the CP might reap the benefit of this enrollment. This reasoning would not explain the magnitude of differences for all forms of inpatient use observed, however. These differences were enormous and more than offset increases in ambulatory care.

The use of encounter data only from three plans raises some question about the completeness of the picture of program effects noted in the evaluation. However, encounter data affect only ambulatory use, and since the major differences were in inpatient use, reporting effects could not account for the findings. The additional information presented regarding access and quality suggests that there appear to have been no adverse consequences associated with the substantial reductions in inpatient use.

Michigan Medicaid Physician Sponsor Plan

Information sources

The principal source documents for this summary were program evaluations conducted by HMA as contracted by the Michigan Department of Social Services for use in the waiver renewal application.* The studies conducted in 1988 and 1989 used the same source data from 1985 and 1986. Findings from the 1986 data analysis were incorporated into the Medicaid program evaluation cited earlier (ORD 1987).

Program description

Michigan offers three alternatives to FFS, freedom-of-choice Medicaid participation. The alternatives correspond to the three prototypes. Enrollment in HMOs (Type 3) is voluntary and has been under way since 1971 with the enrollment of approximately 110,000 in 1989. A small number of beneficiaries are voluntarily enrolled in the CP program, in which health clinics are capitated for nearly all services except inpatient care (Type 2; this plan is described in the previous section). The third program is the PSP, which originated in 1982 in Wayne County (Detroit). The program initially was designed to be mandatory with beneficiaries permitted to opt out only if they enrolled with an HMO or in the CP program. Owing to provider and beneficiary resistance, in practice, participation remained voluntary for several years, including the period covered by the analysis. Officials today portray it as a mandatory enrollment program with approximately 160,000 enrollees.

---

* Health Management Associates, "A Further Analysis of the Michigan Physician Sponsor Plan" (prepared for the Michigan Department of Social Services, Medical Services Administration, Lansing, MI, 1989).

Beneficiaries are enrolled with a participating provider of primary care services who must provide or authorize all services (Type 1). The provider receives FFS payments plus a $3 per month capitation payment for the first 1,000 enrollees, although the mean number of enrollees is less than 100. To expedite enrollment, physicians are permitted to enroll beneficiaries directly through their office, thus supplementing the normal channels for enrollment. Persons not making selection are assigned to a PSP care provider; in the early years, however, switching among PSP physicians was permitted for virtually any reason.

Research method

The 1986 study,* done as part of the MPE, and the 1989 HMA studies are considered more definitive evaluations since program operations were broader in scope by that time. The analyses were multifaceted and examined access, satisfaction, and provider participation as well as cost and use effects. We limit our discussion here to cost and use effects only. The initial analysis proceeded using a before and after comparison group design of continuously eligible beneficiaries, half of whom remained in FFS and half of whom were in the PSP, although there was no attrition in the PSP of persons returning to FFS, as discussed below. The actual sampling strategy was based on prior patterns of use, with three strata: no prior use, medium use, and high use, with use groups being computed for several measures. The appeal of this approach was that it permitted the analysis of differential PCCM effects on these groups, which resulted in interesting and important findings.

The early approach used had some serious problems, in part because prior levels of use were not equal between the groups, that is, high users were underrepresented in the PSP and no users also were underrepresented (because providers enrolled current users). Thus, weights had to be developed to account for prior differences in determining expected effects. Recognizing that enrollment at that stage was voluntary raises the inevitable question of selection bias, which could not be ruled out in the analytical approach used. Another apparent consequence of this strategy was that given regression toward the mean in these continuously eligible groups, one would expect changes at both extremes, which were observed, although the control group was intended to permit removal of this effect. However, because dropping-out patterns suggested that high users were more likely to exit the PSP, the validity of the control-treatment group contrast was confounded. Finally, the analysis looked only at continuously eligible beneficiaries, a group that is not representative of the eligible population as a whole. Other groups such as newborns and persons with obstetrical deliveries and catastrophic expenses were separated and, in some cases, analyzed separately to prevent the contamination of the basic analysis.

The later analyses used cross-sectional contrasts of large groups of enrollees versus nonenrollees and calculated use and cost levels for FFS persons adjusting

---

* Michigan Department of Social Services, ''The Impact of the Physician Primary Sponsor Plan on the Medicaid Program in Michigan'' (Lansing, MI: Office of Planning, Budget, and Evaluation, 1986).

for age and gender groupings. These levels were then applied to the groupings among PSP enrollees to produce estimated levels of use and expenditures that could be compared to actual expenditures. Although the sample sizes were very large (36,000 PSP enrollees), the cross-sectional nature of the analysis could not control on a person-level basis for other contributory factors, including prior levels of use.

The analytical approach used claims-based data to examine cost and use effects. (In an FFS PCCM program, claims are a reliable data source.) The focus was on individuals with some use, since the evaluators contended that the impact of PCCM could only be experienced if individuals were using some services. The analysis also produced separate estimates by selected age groups that could reveal the relative merits of targeting the intervention. The basic strategy involved calculating actual FFS rates of cost and use in the comparison group and then applying these to the age and gender strata of the enrolled populations to produce expected versus actual expenditures. Multivariate techniques were not used to equate individuals for the analysis.

The later analysis (1989) introduced some new approaches to reanalyzing the data and to calculating cost savings, but the validity of these approaches seems doubtful. They included assertions that improved family planning by PSP physicians reduced obstetrical costs; they imputed uniform obstetric hospital costs when it appeared that PSP physicians used higher-cost facilities; and they claimed that a portion of the PCCM case management fee should represent service expansion (availability for phone calls, etc.) rather than an additional administrative cost.

Findings

An important general finding reported in the earlier PSP analysis was that with respect to the low, medium, and high user groups, a distinctive pattern was evident. Use and costs increased slightly for the low users, decreased sharply for the high users, and decreased by a smaller amount for the medium users when compared with costs for FFS beneficiaries. Looking at expected use experience of enrollees with some use, as based on FFS experience in the comparison group, the following patterns were observed. Physician visits were higher for PSP enrollees (4.4 versus 4.1), emergency department use was slightly lower (0.35 versus 0.44), ancillary use was mixed, and prescription use was higher (10.1 versus 9.06). Inpatient use was lower (415 days per 1,000 versus 581 days per 1,000).

A parallel analysis was performed for persons with obstetric delivery stays during the period, approximately 1,000 persons. Physician visits were slightly higher than expected (7.2 versus 6.6), emergency department visits were slightly lower, ancillary use was unchanged, and prescription use slightly higher. Inpatient use was slightly lower for obstetrical purposes, but nonobstetric admissions were sharply lower.

The overall estimates of cost impact were computed for persons with expenses using actual versus expected cost estimates. For nonobstetric PSP enrollees, the actual cost ($753) was approximately 12 percent less than the expected cost of $858. There was virtually no difference for obstetric cases ($4,878 versus $4,843), although as noted above, this result was before the evaluators standardized the hospital cost component to adjust for the fact that PSP physicians appeared to be using higher-cost hospitals. This adjustment resulted in a difference of about $250, or about 5 percent (i.e., PSP enrollee costs were adjusted downward by about 5 percent).

In aggregating the findings resulting from the 1989 cost impact, including the adding back of case management fees and administrative costs, the evaluators estimated net cost savings to be approximately 4.1 percent, which was approximately half of the 8.0 percent savings reported in the earlier analysis. The evaluators provided a detailed account of why they believed this estimate was highly conservative. They asserted that true savings for the analysis period more likely were 10 percent and could have been as high as 15 to 16 percent.

Assessment

The scope and depth of the evaluations performed on the PSP are impressive, if rather seriously out of date given that the data being evaluated were from 1986. The segmentation of program effects by low, medium, and high users remains a valuable contribution that has highly important targeting implications. Specifically, it suggests the effectiveness of the program might have been twofold: improving access for low users and curbing excessive use among high users, a conclusion amplified in the evaluation with respect to children and adults. The level of detail available on types of utilization is also impressive, even though this variable was only reported for those with some use. Missing are proportions of populations that had no use, which would also be highly informative.

The age of the data here is particularly problematic since the program evaluated in 1986 was still more voluntary than mandatory (or at least not sufficiently mandatory that it was clear who would be in and who would not yet be enrolled). This problem means the findings are vulnerable to selection bias, which appears consistent with some of the findings, although in general the bias might have been adverse for providers and thus might have had a conservative effect on the cost savings estimates. Moreover, the more clearly mandatory nature of the program today raises questions whether the 1990 program effects can be expected to be similar. Also missing in this analysis is a discussion of how those persons in the PSP might have differed from HMO and CP enrollees.

The analysis did not use person-level models or statistical tests to evaluate the significance of differences. This is particularly of interest since several of the findings were relatively small in magnitude and potentially attributable to differences that have not been controlled for. Finally, as noted above, several judgments made about the cost estimates in the 1989 projects appear somewhat arbitrary.

Minnesota Prepaid Demonstration Project in Hennepin and Dakota Counties

Information sources

The Minnesota program was studied as part of the Medicaid Competition Demonstrations. However, it was not one of the programs for which a full-scale cost and use analysis was performed, partly because of the unavailability of expected secondary data. As a result, the data for the analysis came from (1) two consumer surveys, one done prior to implementation in 1986 and the other after implementation in 1988,* and (2) multiyear case studies, also done under the RTI contract.

Program description

Minnesota chose to participate in the MCDs to test prepaid programs in urban (Hennepin), suburban (Dakota), and rural (Itasca) counties. There was a prolonged delay in starting the Hennepin and Dakota county programs because of provider and other resistance, despite the widespread acceptance of HMOs in the marketplace. Ultimately, the program was a novel one in that it introduced an experimental design into the demonstration. Thirty-five percent of essentially all eligible Medicaid beneficiaries were randomly assigned to be enrolled in seven (later six) PHPs in the greater Minneapolis area. Once informed of their assignment to the program, these beneficiaries were provided with information on each of the plans so that they could select one that would be their case manager and source of care.

The basic design of the program was mandatory enrollment in HMOs that, in return for capitation payments, were to provide or arrange all services for members (Type 3). An elaborate set of rates was developed to cover the broad spectrum of beneficiaries who were to be enrolled. Among the participating plans were three large, well-established HMOs; three smaller plans—two of which were launched chiefly to permit participation; and the Blue Cross/Blue Shield (BC/BS) plan. The BC/BS plan, which had the largest enrollment at one time, dropped out in January 1988, and its enrollees were redistributed across the remaining six plans. At the same time, the state also chose to exempt the disabled from participation in the program. The findings reported here pertain only to AFDC beneficiaries.

Research method

The original evaluation design for the program was to exploit the random assignment in the program design by tracking panels of enrollees and nonenrollees via consumer experience surveys over the year before and the first year of the demonstration. An initial survey was fielded in 1986 in Minnesota to permit this evaluation to be done. Moreover, the design also anticipated having pseudoclaims available from the capitated providers. Neither of the aims was fully met. Slippage in implementation frustrated the ability to track panels of enrollees and nonenrollees, and the plans failed to submit pseudoclaims in a reliable, usable form.

To accommodate the former difficulty, the second-wave survey—which could only be done after two years—comprised three subgroups. One group was a panel of those persons still eligible and enrolled in a plan for whom pre- and postenrollment data would be available. The second group was a representative sample of enrollees in 1988 who were not in the panel, and the third group was a represen-

---

* Research Triangle Institute (RTI), *Evaluation of the Medicaid Competition Demonstrations: The Minnesota Consumer Surveys*, HCFA Contract No. 500-83-0050 (Research Triangle Park, NC: Research Triangle Institute, 1989).

tative sample of nonenrollees. This design thus allowed before and after contrasts (without a comparison group) and a cross-sectional analysis of enrollees and nonenrollees. The consumer survey conducted via personal interview had high response rates among all groups, all of which were stratified random samples.

The consumer survey incorporated an extensive set of questions on background, resources, attitudes, health status and behaviors, and self-reported inpatient and ambulatory use. The use data relied on three-month recall periods for ambulatory use and one-year recall for inpatient use. No cost data were collected with this instrument. The 1989 RTI analysis presented descriptive bivariate statistics that compared the experience of the various contrast groups. In addition, multivariate analyses of use were conducted controlling for person-level characteristics. Satisfaction and access also were analyzed extensively with these same data.

Findings

The findings for the evaluation of program effects are available for AFDC adults and children (as well as for SSI beneficiaries) from both the panel and the cross-sectional analyses. No significant differences were found between enrollees and nonenrollees (or between enrollees before and during the demonstration) in utilization measures examining ambulatory use with and without physician participation, emergency department use, or inpatient use. Prescription use was not reported. It is possible that the relatively small sample sizes weaken the ability to detect differences, should these differences be small. The bivariate analyses suggest that this problem may have been the case for emergency department visits, which were slightly lower for enrollees, and ambulatory visits, which were slightly higher. Nonetheless, these differences were minor. The lack of differences is especially notable given random assignment to the program, which prevented self-selection bias.

Several reasons for lack of observed program effects were advanced. The most plausible of these is that access to care was already high among the eligible population and prepayment was so prevalent in the Minneapolis market that substantial changes in patterns of use were unlikely. As an indication of the stability experienced in the program, more than half of the AFDC beneficiaries (and two-thirds of the SSI beneficiaries) enrolled with their prior usual source of care. It is this "business as usual" phenomenon that might explain why, for example, emergency department visits did not decline as they had in all of the other Medicaid demonstrations.

Assessment

The experimental design feature of random assignment is an impressive feature of this particular demonstration program. Also, the two-component analysis, panel and cross-sectional, is a strength of the evaluation performed. The fact that neither analysis detected significant impacts on use supports the view that the intervention had little effect. However, the small sample sizes diminish the ability to detect significant differences, and the inclusion of a panel of never-enrolled persons would have improved the design substantially. The use of self-reported use has potential limitations, although the conventions for recall used were common and acceptable. Given the severe underreporting of pseudoclaims, self-reported use was the only available data source. Unfortunately, no cost data were available.

Minnesota Prepaid Medicaid Demonstration in Itasca County

The Itasca County program was studied as part of the Medicaid Competition Demonstrations but was not one of the programs for which a full-scale cost-and-use analysis was performed. Two case studies that incorporated program-provided data on performance were done by Lewin/ICF, an RTI subcontractor, and were the principal sources for this assessment.* The Lewin/RTI second case study was dated October 1988.

Program description

Minnesota chose to participate in the MCDs to test prepaid programs in urban (Hennepin), suburban (Dakota), and rural (Itasca) counties. Itasca is a relatively remote northern county that had some prior experience with prepayment in the early 1980s under a block grant program with the state. In 1985 the county agreed to act as an HIO to offer a prepaid Medicaid program to approximately 3,400 AFDC, SSI, and General Assistance (GA) beneficiaries. As an inducement to participate, the state agreed to pay half of the county's 5 percent Medicaid share. The state paid the county a capitation rate of 90 percent of expected FFS for AFDC beneficiaries and 95 percent for aged, blind, and disabled patients (blind and disabled patients later were dropped from the prepaid program).

The program is administered by a county task force that includes provider representatives. A contract was signed with the Blue Cross HMO subsidiary to process claims, perform utilization reviews, and produce MIS reports. The HIO entered into contracts with PCPs, dentists, and pharmacists, who became a primary care team that provided or authorized all beneficiary services. In return, the at-risk physicians and hospitals initially were paid 90 percent of their usual, customary, and reasonable fees. This amount later was reduced to 75 percent, with the remainder retained in a withholding fund (Type 2). Utilization review controls initially were relatively weak but were strengthened as the program experienced financial pressures. Some effects of this strengthening were noted. As in many programs with the HIO structure, considerable debate occurred with the state about the

---

* Research Triangle Institute (RTI), *Evaluation of the Medicaid Competition Demonstrations: Case Study Reports,* HCFA Contract No. 500-83-0050 (Research Triangle Park, NC: Research Triangle Institute, 1989).

appropriateness of the rate-setting methodology, including the use of 1982 as the rate base.

The program was highly regarded by many providers as an attempt to customize the local Medicaid program, although some provider groups felt adversely affected. The hospitals felt the payment method in Itasca was not as favorable as the one they would have experienced in the statewide per diem method used elsewhere in Minnesota. Dentists felt that payments should be made out of a separate risk pool rather than out of the medical pool.

Research method

The analysis done by program managers in Itasca County is the only available study of program effects and was reported in the second case study. It was a descriptive analysis for which no prior program experience or control group experience was reported. Because it involved primary care gatekeeping with a risk-sharing arrangement, the reported findings cannot be attributed to either feature individually. The availability of three years of utilization data does provide a longitudinal picture of program effects.

Findings

The data available were provided by HMO-Minnesota based on cost and utilization reports. They included information on inpatient use, physician visits, emergency department visits, and prescription use (cost) as well as other measures. Between year 1 and year 3, inpatient use declined from 742 days per 1,000 to 589 days, or 20.6 percent. Office visits increased from 3.5 to 4.0, or 14.3 percent. Emergency department visits increased from 0.14 per enrollee to 0.17, or 21.4 percent, over the three years. Prescription drug costs declined by 8.3 percent from year 1 to year 2, the only years for which these data were available. Unfortunately, no summary measure of cost experience per enrollee was reported. Given the capitation payment arrangement between the state and the HIO, the state was guaranteed savings. However, the HIO reported substantial losses ($400,000 in the first year of operation). This loss led to a redoubling of utilization review efforts and to the petitioning of the state to reevaluate the method for calculating the capitation rate. This request was unsuccessful and raised questions about the continued support of providers and, thus, the long-term viability of the program.

Assessment

Even though this is a small and highly idiosyncratic program whose generalizability is very limited, it does provide a picture of the potential applicability of PCCM programs to rural areas. Unfortunately, no rigorous evaluation of the program was conducted, although the case study findings of lower inpatient use and higher physician use are not inconsistent with those reported in other Type 2 programs. In the absence of preprogram data or a legitimate comparison group, many potentially confounding factors cannot be ruled out.

Missouri Physician Sponsors Plan

Information sources

The main sources for this study were RTI's MCD evaluation and various publications using data accumulated during that evaluation, including Hurley, Paul, and Freund.*

Program description

The Missouri PHP program was established in 1983 and continues to the present, along with the Physician Sponsors Plan (PSP), as the Medicaid program for AFDC beneficiaries in Jackson County (Kansas City). The PSP evolved as an alternative to the PHP programs. It was designed to permit a group of primary care physicians who would be paid fee-for-service with a nominal case management fee to function as gatekeepers (Type 1). These 50-plus physicians had traditionally provided a substantial amount of care to the Medicaid population and feared that the conversion of the Medicaid program to prepayment would sever longstanding relationships and adversely affect their practices.

The state accommodated these physicians by enabling them to formally enroll into their (now gatekeeping) practice approximately 3,000 to 4,000 beneficiaries who were already receiving the bulk of their care from these physicians. These physicians were not required to accept randomly assigned, nonselecting beneficiaries, as were the PHPs. Although a detailed analysis of selection bias among plans found no significant evidence of bias, enrollees in the PSP were more likely to have a prior relationship and selected their PSP in the interest of sustaining this relationship.

Research method

This program enrolled beneficiaries with a PCP-gatekeeper who continued to be paid FFS. Because in nearly every case these persons were already seeing their PCP before enrollment, the program presented a special opportunity to examine the experience of persons going into a gatekeeping program without having the prior relationship disrupted.

The general analytical approach used in the RTI study to assess cost and use effects was a quasi-experimental design with a before and after nonequivalent comparison group. Data for claims for stratified random samples of approximately 2,000 children and 1,000 adults for the demonstration county and a comparison county (St. Louis) were extracted for the year prior to the demonstration and the first year of the demonstration. Person-level utilization cost files were built for each

---

* Research Triangle Institute (RTI), *Evaluation of the Medicaid Competition Demonstrations: Case Study Reports,* HCFA Contract No. 500-83-0050 (Research Triangle Park, NC: Research Triangle Institute, 1989); R. E. Hurley, J. Paul, and D. Freund, "Going into Gatekeeping: An Empirical Assessment," *Quality Review Bulletin* 15, no. 10 (1989): 306–14.

person in the samples for use in developing mean levels of cost and use. Using data from eligibility files for sample members, evaluators developed multivariate models of use for several use measures employing the RAND two-part model of use: probability of use and use for users only.

Measures of use were available for inpatient admissions and days; physician visits by specialty; emergency department use; ancillary use; care concentration; and, though not previously reported, prescription use. The analysis of program effects assessed the impact of being the demonstration site in the demonstration year after controlling for a number of person-level variables.

The principal evaluation of this program compared the entire Jackson County demonstration to the program in St. Louis County, which meant including the FFS gatekeeping (Type 1) PSP with the PHPs. Subsequent detailed analyses compared the two programs to examine how the PHPs might have differed from the PSP. The analysis of the PSP discussed these differences in greater detail. A special analysis file was created to look at a panel of beneficiaries eligible in both the pre- and post-years who could be observed "going into gatekeeping."* Since the method of payment was not altered, the claims data in the before and after years were comparable. Similarly, because the same persons were analyzed, covariates were not needed.

Findings

The results of the analyses are available for adults and children in terms of use and cost effects. There was some evidence of reductions in inpatient use for children (percent with a stay), which was an artifact of newborns who could only appear in the initial year. The probability of an emergency department use was 50 percent lower for children and 35 to 40 percent lower for adults compared to the prior year's level of use.

Physician visit effects suggested reductions in specialty visits for children, especially in visits for users (62 percent), while the effects were similar but smaller for adults (35 percent). Primary care visits for children were virtually unchanged, while for adults there was a compensating increase in primary care visits so that total physician visits actually rose for them. More care was concentrated with the gatekeeper PCP. Prescription use (which was not capitated) was slightly lower (less than 10 percent) for children and somewhat lower for adults (15 to 20 percent).

The cost analysis indicated there were no significant reductions in costs in the first year of the program for adults and children. Although differences were noted for children, the amount of variation was too great to ascertain whether such differences were due to chance. Adult expenditures were nearly identical ($613 and $607).

Assessment

The before and after panel analysis was a straightforward attempt to see how converting one's prior usual source of care to a formal gatekeeper affected use and costs.

---

* Hurley, Paul, and Freund, "Going into Gatekeeping."

Since the method of payment changed for some and remained as FFS for others, the analyses were not confounded by underreporting. The panel analysis obviated the need to control for other variables.

The main limitations lie in the small, opportunistic sample available to perform this analysis. The sample would have been too small to detect significant differences unless they were sizable. This was a function of the fact that the PSP study was a by-product of the larger Jackson County–wide comparison to St. Louis County. For example, the consumer survey analysis did not detect differences between the PSP and other plans when using self-reported measures of use. The other important caveat about the findings regarding the PSP is that almost by definition, the enrollees were being gatekept by their prior usual source of care. Most Type 1 programs are not so structured, as many (if not most) of the enrollee-gatekeeper relationships begin with the introduction of the gatekeeper program.

Despite these limitations, the experience of the PSP program as reported in the analysis is informative regarding the impact of Type 1 programs. The panel design remains one of the few to explicitly track the effects of the entry into gatekeeping.

Missouri Prepaid Health Plan Program

Information sources

The main sources for this study were RTI's MCD evaluation* and various publications using data accumulated during the evaluation.†

Program description

The Missouri PHP program was established in 1983 and continues to the present, along with the PSP, as the Medicaid program for AFDC beneficiaries in Jackson County (Kansas City). In the PHP program four (originally five) primary care organizations are paid capitation payments for virtually all Medicaid-covered services for beneficiaries, who are required to enroll with one of the four plans (Type 3). There are approximately 16,000 persons in the plans. Approximately 3,000 to 4,000 patients are enrolled in the PSP, which is an FFS gatekeeper alternative (described above).

---

* Research Triangle Institute (RTI), *Evaluation of the Medicaid Competition Demonstrations: Integrative Final Report,* HCFA Contract No. 500-83-0050 (Research Triangle Park, NC: Research Triangle Institute, 1989).

† For example, R. E. Hurley, D. Freund, and D. Taylor, "Emergency Room Use and Primary Care Case Management: Evidence from Four Medicaid Demonstration Programs," *American Journal of Public Health* 79, no. 7 (1989): 843–46; and R. E. Hurley, D. Freund, and D. Taylor, "Gatekeeping the Emergency Room: Impact of a Medicaid Primary Care Case Management Program," *Health Care Management Review* 14, no. 2 (1989): 63–71.

The four existing plans include an IPA-model HMO, two neighborhood health centers, and one large public hospital outpatient department. The fifth plan also was a hospital outpatient department, but it subsequently dropped out and most of its enrollees joined the other hospital plan. Of the four plans, only the IPA was a true HMO, established as a subsidiary of a preexisting HMO to enable physicians to serve Medicaid beneficiaries. The other plans had no prior experience with prepaid programs. While the hospital plan enrolled approximately 40 percent of beneficiaries, a detailed analysis of selection bias among plans found no significant evidence of bias. The plans all received the same capitation payment with one rate for adults and one for children. The limited number of plans and corresponding large enrollments created sufficiently large risk pools for most losses, and the state had catastrophic stop-loss pools for high-risk and high-cost deliveries.

The IPA pays physicians by FFS and withholds, whereas the institutional providers have salaried physicians. It is not clear how much individual assignment to physicians occurred in the health centers and outpatient departments, but it probably was less than in the IPA, which used a gatekeeper system.

Research method

This program enrolled beneficiaries into PHPs that received capitation for the full scope of covered services (Type 3). As such, the program introduced both PCCM and capitation. The analyses performed did not examine these components separately, although interplan analyses were performed.

The general analytical approach used in the RTI study to assess cost and use effects was a quasi-experimental design with a before and after nonequivalent comparison group. Data used were from claims for stratified random samples of approximately 2,000 children and 1,000 adults for the demonstration county and a comparison county (St. Louis) for the year prior to the demonstration and the first year of the demonstration. Person-level utilization cost files were built for each person in the samples for use in developing mean levels of cost and use. Using data from eligibility files for sample members, evaluators developed multivariate models of use for several use measures employing the RAND two-part model of use: probability of use and use for users only.

Measures of use were available for inpatient admissions and days, physician visits by specialty, emergency department use, ancillary use, care concentration, and—though not previously reported—prescription use. The analysis of program effects assessed the impact of being the demonstration site in the demonstration year after controlling for a number of person-level variables. A potential problem, given the capitation payment, is the underreporting of encounters. Providers were required to submit pseudoclaims for these services, but detailed analysis suggests that underreporting did occur and was probably not uniform across all plans. The IPA plan apparently had the most underreporting.

The principal evaluation of this program compared the entire Jackson County demonstration to the program in St. Louis County, which meant including the FFS gatekeeping (Type 1) PSP with the PHPs. Subsequent detailed analyses compared the two programs to examine how the PHPs might have differed from the PSP. The analysis of the PSP discussed these differences in greater detail.

In addition to this cost and use analysis with claims data, the Missouri data also were analyzed via a Medicaid consumer survey with AFDC beneficiaries and via a quality-of-care study; both studies employed St. Louis County as the comparison site. While highly informative on a number of program features, the findings from the claims data analysis are viewed as the more definitive with respect to cost and use effects.

Findings

The results of the analyses are available for adults and children in terms of use and cost effects. There was some evidence of reductions in inpatient use for children (percent with a stay), which could have been an artifact of oversampling of persons with two years of eligibility since newborns could only appear in the initial year.

Days per thousand were lower by about 12 percent for adults. Probability of an emergency department visit was 35 percent lower for children and 44 percent lower for adults compared to the prior year's level of use. A notable interplan finding was that the hospital outpatient department plans had no reduction in emergency department use corresponding to reductions in the IPA and the neighborhood health centers, suggesting that they used the emergency department for after-hour coverage.

Physician visit reductions were limited. Because the specialty of physicians among the institutional providers could not be determined from the pseudoclaims, primary care versus specialist analyses are unreliable. Ancillary use was lower by between 25 and 35 percent but this could have been due in part to underreporting. Prescription use (which was not capitated) was lower by between 15 and 30 percent for children and adults (although this reduction was smaller in the PSP).

The cost analysis indicated an interesting anomaly of prepayment. The capitation payments were slightly lower than they were during the previous year ($731 versus $751) for adults and slightly higher ($325 to $338) for children. However, given reductions in the levels of use, the FFS equivalent payment was $415 for adults and $208 for children (in part due to underreporting). The state in effect paid rates 22 percent higher than it should have. Rates subsequently were adjusted downward by 19 percent in the following year. The anomaly is that if utilization were to fall sharply, rates based on prior-year levels of use would appear to be excessive. This effect was especially pronounced in Missouri since the St. Louis County comparison site experienced a real decline in expenditures between the years before and after the demonstration.

The interplan analyses among the providers in Kansas City revealed no significant differences other than the lack of effect on emergency department use in the hospital plans.

Assessment

Like all the MCD studies, this analysis generally is well done, with large samples from claims data in the context of a good research design. However, the underreporting issue is a problem in Missouri, except for the PSP, which continued to pay FFS. The use of a comparison site enabled some control for history effects. Program maturation is a problem here, especially since this program has now been in operation for four years since the analysis of it was conducted. There is some reason to be concerned about the true comparability of St. Louis County to Jackson County (Kansas City), given the former's much larger size and greater urban character.

Like the Santa Barbara County (California) study, the results in Missouri are well triangulated by the availability of consumer survey findings and a quality-of-care study, both of which help to provide a comprehensive picture of a primary care management program in Medicaid. The multiple participating plans provide opportunities to study several other features of the program regarding plan choice, and also the ability of existing institutional providers to convert to prepayment when faced with the opportunity or the need.

Nevada Enrolled Health Plan

Information sources

The principal sources of information for this assessment were the MPE,* which included Nevada, and the most recent state waiver documentation, including cost savings estimates for fiscal years 1989 and 1990.

Program description

Nevada initiated a Medicaid PCCM program in November 1983. The project was a unique enterprise in that it was jointly offered with the University of Nevada–Las Vegas (UNLV) and the University of Nevada–Reno (UNR) family practice departments. The basic design was intended to enroll Medicaid beneficiaries in each city (primarily AFDC, but others were permitted to participate) voluntarily with the family practice departments at the two university medical schools. The goals were to provide cost containment, continuity, and a flow of patients and dollars to the medical school departments.

In principle, beneficiaries were to enroll with specified faculty members and residents who would provide or authorize all covered services (in practice, however, enrollment has been with the clinic rather than with individual physicians). The family practice departments are paid a capitation rate for all ambulatory services, including physician, emergency department visits, laboratory work and x-rays, and prescriptions. Other services, including referral care and inpatient care, are paid

---

* Office of Research and Demonstrations (ORD), *Medicaid Program Evaluation: Final Report*, Report No. MPE 9.2, eds. J. Holahan, J. Bell, and G. S. Adler (Baltimore, MD: Health Care Financing Administration, 1987).

on an FFS basis and have to be authorized even though most of the care is provided by university-affiliated providers. This program is basically Type 2, but because gatekeepers are salaried faculty and residents, they are not at direct financial risk, like Type 3 programs or PHPs (which receive capitation for the full scope of services). The capitation rate is set based on FFS experience for the unenrolled populations in the two cities. Separate rates are determined for Reno and Las Vegas.

In this voluntary program, enrollment is achieved by inducing individuals to join. Enrollment has been slow, with approximately 4,000 enrollees in February 1991 out of a potential pool of 30,000 in the two urban counties. Some problems have been encountered in marketing the program. The new program also has faced some resistance from PCPs unaffiliated with the medical schools who have lost patients who chose to enroll. To induce enrollment, copayments are waived, as are state limits on numbers of physician visits. It is also believed that the 24-hour availability condition for UNLV and UNR family practice clinic physicians is appealing to prospective enrollees.

Research method

No detailed evaluation of this program has been conducted in terms of impact on cost and use. The MPE relied on state waiver application data, and this is the source of the most recent program experience. Program quality audits have been completed by departmental staff, and the sites are required to submit encounter data despite being paid on a capitation basis for most ambulatory services. As noted below, there does not appear to be a serious underreporting problem in the University of Nevada utilization data. Comparative data from nonenrollees in both cities were included for contrast.

Cost estimates also are presented only by eligibility category, age, and gender. These estimates allow one to examine which groups are responsible for savings—i.e., expenditures for beneficiaries in PCCM were less than for FFS nonenrollees. Because no investigation of selection bias has been performed, it is not known whether the lower-than-expected expenditures in PCCM are caused by favorable selection or by something else. Moreover, the payment method could conceivably underpay the University of Nevada schools substantially compared to costs, or compared to expected use for enrollees; but the special status and goals of the program might accept such nonmarket rates.

Findings

The savings in 1989 and 1990 approached $1.5 million with about two-thirds of the savings in Las Vegas and one-third in Reno in both years. The savings in AFDC were due primarily to children less than one year old and women of childbearing age. This result suggests that the capitation rate, which was uniform for adults and for children, might systematically underpay for obstetrical and delivery care rendered to the enrolled populations. In other words, a rate unadjusted for pregnancy might overpay for nonpregnant and underpay for pregnant women. Likewise, for newborns, a fixed rate set on expected use might underpay for well-child care.

Utilization findings also present a somewhat inconclusive picture. Hospital days in Las Vegas (281 versus 740) and Reno (337 versus 865) were dramatically lower for enrollees versus nonenrollees. This could be an indication of either favorable selection bias or improved care management. Notably, physician visits and prescription use were higher in both sites relative to those for the comparison groups. Physician visits were up by over 30 percent in both sites. Prescriptions were 100 percent higher in Reno and about 50 percent higher in Las Vegas.

Laboratory use was markedly higher in the PCCM groups, although the FFS rates were questionably low, suggesting that there might be a problem with the data. Emergency department use was dramatically lower for enrollees. In Las Vegas the rate of visits was 35 per 100 versus 104, and in Reno the enrollee rate was 21 per 100 versus 83. These findings suggest that effective gatekeeping of the emergency department was occurring. The quality audits performed in both clinic settings suggest generally good performance. It appears, however, that both programs relied more on institutional case management than on individual physician case management.

Assessment

The design and operation of this particular program are virtually unique among PCCM programs, given the special medical school affiliation. Particularly notable is the interest in the schools' participation to ensure financial and legislative support, which suggests that they might maintain participation even if the payment arrangements were not entirely favorable. The cost savings projections suggest that this might be the case.

The analysis done to support the waiver was very limited. Most significantly, there was no assessment of selection bias. Because the program is voluntary and has enrolled fewer than 15 percent of potential enrollees, it is highly likely that enrollment is not entirely random. Consequently, the asserted savings are not attributable to an operational feature of the program. The fact that the savings are due to a limited number of beneficiary groups suggests that the capitation rate might not be adequately calibrated. On the other hand, the acceptance of the rate by the University of Nevada system might be the best indication of its appropriateness.

Regarding the utilization findings, these effects generally are consistent with what might occur in this type of design with this type of provider population. Again, the very low inpatient use is surprising since the medical schools are not at risk for inpatient use—suggesting bias in enrollment. In sum, then, these findings have only marginal usefulness.

New Jersey Medicaid Personal Physician Plan

Information sources

The primary sources for this study were the MCD evaluation* and various publications using data accumulated during the evaluation.†

Program description

The New Jersey Medicaid Personal Physician (MP) program was established in 1984 as a voluntary PCCM gatekeeper program in which PCPs (physicians and health centers) were paid capitation for primary care services and given opportunities to participate in shared savings in referral accounts (Type 2). Inpatient care was excluded from the referral accounts and continued to be paid by diagnosis-related groups (DRGs).

The program was intended to be phased in until it was available statewide to persons wishing to enroll voluntarily. It was offered initially to rural counties in northwest New Jersey, but beneficiary interest exceeded the capacity of physicians willing to participate. Eventually the program was extended to two urban counties—Essex (Newark) and Camden—but enrollment proceeded very slowly and never exceeded 12,000 over the life of the program. Enrollment was so problematic that the state eventually allowed physicians to directly enroll patients already in their practices into the prepayment program. In addition, the state waived the downside risk in the first year of the program to encourage providers to participate.

Because the program was voluntary and providers had an opportunity to selectively convert some of their FFS patients to capitation, a careful analysis of selection bias was conducted in this program. No evidence of significant selection bias was detected, insofar as indication that the capitation rates were excessive or insufficient. However, it does appear that persons who did enroll had slightly higher previous year expenses. This could have been because, for physicians to enroll through their practices, the patients had to already be using some services. Thus, nonusers were less likely to be enrolled.

The program ultimately was discontinued because of its inability to expand at the desired rate and because of some difficulties the state experienced in complying with the requirements of the demonstration waiver mandates. It was replaced with a state-run HMO, the Garden State Health Plan.

---

* Research Triangle Institute (RTI), *Evaluation of the Medicaid Competition Demonstrations: Integrative Final Report*, HCFA Contract No. 500-83-0050 (Research Triangle Park, NC: Research Triangle Institute, 1989).

† For example, R. E. Hurley, D. Freund, and D. Taylor, "Emergency Room Use and Primary Care Case Management: Evidence from Four Medicaid Demonstration Programs," *American Journal of Public Health* 79, no. 7 (1989): 843–46; and R. E. Hurley, D. Freund, and D. Taylor, "Gatekeeping and Emergency Room: Impact of a Medicaid Primary Care Case Management Program," *Health Care Management Review* 14, no. 2 (1989): 63–71.

Research method

This program enrolled beneficiaries with PCPs who received capitation for primary care services. Funds were deposited into an individual referral account to cover all remaining services except for inpatient care. Gatekeepers were allowed to participate in savings associated with the residuals in the referral account. As such, this plan introduced both primary care gatekeeping and capitation, and the analyses performed did not examine these components separately.

The general analytical approach used in the RTI study to assess cost and use effects was a quasi-experimental design with a before and after nonequivalent comparison group. Data were extracted from claims files for stratified random samples of approximately 2,000 children and 1,000 adults for the demonstration county (Camden) and for a comparison county (Atlantic) for the year prior to the demonstration and the first year of the demonstration. Person-level utilization cost files were built for each person in the samples for use in developing mean levels of cost and use. Using data from eligibility files for sample members, evaluators developed multivariate models of use for several use measures employing the RAND two-part model of use: probability of use and use for users only.

Measures of use were available for inpatient admissions and days, physician visits by specialty, emergency department use, ancillary use, care concentration, and prescription use. The analysis of program effects assessed the impact of being the demonstration county in the demonstration year after controlling for a number of person-level variables. A potential problem, given the capitation payment, is underreporting of encounters. Providers were required to submit pseudoclaims for these services, but detailed analysis suggests that underreporting did occur in primary care services given the program design and the method of payment.

In New Jersey, the basic analytical approach was modified to include in the analysis a substantial sample of individuals who had continuous eligibility in both years, some of whom enrolled voluntarily and others of whom did not enroll. This supplemental sample/panel design was chosen to conduct the selection bias study. It also was used to perform tests of cost and use effects after controlling for levels of use in the previous year. These findings also are reported below.

Findings

The results of the analyses are available for adults and children in terms of use and cost effects, and for the full sample and the panel of continuously eligible persons. No significant inpatient effects were detected for any group in any analysis, which is consistent with the exclusion of inpatient care from financial risk-bearing by the primary care gatekeeper. However, emergency department use was sharply lower for adults (43 percent) and for children (37 percent) in the overall analysis. Rates for children and adults were very similar when evaluators controlled for prior-year emergency department use in the panel study. Small reductions in physician use were observed for enrollees, but because increases were observed for nonenrollees, and given the nature of the analysis done, these differences were significant.

The reductions in physician visits showed a net effect of sharp reductions in specialist visits and, at least for adults, an increase in primary care visits. While there was evidence of underreporting of physician visits in New Jersey, this would only occur for primary care services since referral physicians remained under FFS. Consequently, the inverse relationship/substitution effect of primary care for specialty care appears to be a valid finding. Ancillary use was sharply lower but also was highly susceptible to underreporting since the primary care capitation payment covered basic laboratory and x-ray services. More care was concentrated with the primary care gatekeeper. Though not tested in the multivariate models, no pattern of change in prescription use was noted.

The cost effects in New Jersey indicate several things. On average, previous year expenses were higher for children (355 versus 277) and for adults (1,041 versus 882), suggesting that enrollees tended to be sicker than nonenrollees. The demonstration year FFS equivalent costs for children and adults were lower than the previous year costs for enrollees, as would be expected given the reductions in use reported above (though underreporting may account for this phenomenon). The multivariate analysis of costs revealed that there were no statistically significant effects on costs for children. This means that the capitation rate paid was approximately equal to what the expected expenditure under FFS would have been given the cost experience of the nonenrollees and controlling for person-level characteristics. For adults, the expected expenditure was actually 11 percent higher than for the actual FFS payment; this amount was statistically significant.

Assessment

Like the other MCD studies, this analysis generally was well-done, with large samples from claims data in the context of a good research design. Using a panel of continuously eligible persons and controlling for prior levels of use further strengthened the analysis of utilization effects. On the other hand, the underreporting issue is a problem for analyzing primary care service use in New Jersey, although the fact that it diminishes but does not eliminate the substitution of primary care for specialty care suggests this was a robust effect. The use of a comparison group of nonenrollees to complete the analysis and to probe for selection bias evidence (not found) are additional positives for this study.

The New Jersey program was a small, slowly implemented one, in part because of its voluntary nature, which, in turn, inhibited its rapid expansion. Thus, the program's generalizability is limited. Likewise, the use of gatekeepers to recruit enrollees and the dilution of program features (dropping risk-sharing in the first year of participation to increase provider participation) raise questions about program coherence and integrity. However, it was the only voluntary program extensively studied in the MCDs.

Erie County (New York) Physician Case Management Program (Children)

Information sources

The only source of information for this program was the Report to the Legislature on the Implementation of the Medicaid Reform Act of 1984, prepared by the New York State Department of Health.*

Program description

State background. The state of New York has engaged in Medicaid managed care initiatives for many years. Until 1984, virtually all this activity involved the enrollment of beneficiaries in HMOs. Most sites offered enrollment on a voluntary basis—with the exception of Monroe County, which was one of the sites for the MCDs (unfortunately, no cost and use data became available from that program). In 1984, new legislation was passed to promote the expansion of other managed care models to accelerate enrollment, which was constrained by insufficient participation of established HMOs.

Two new models were promoted:

1. Beneficiaries were enrolled with primary care organizations such as neighborhood health clinics that could receive capitation for the full scope of beneficiary services and function as a PHP. A number of such programs were under way, primarily in urban areas. The state subsidized the development of these programs and continues to work toward building capacity and enrollment. Current enrollment is small and only descriptive findings are available.
2. The other model introduced primary care networks that employ physician case management with some degree of financial risk sharing. Total enrollment in all programs reached 46,000 by the end of 1989.

Erie County program. The Erie County Physician Case Management Program 1 (PCMP-1) is a PCCM program for children patterned after the Suffolk County (Long Island) Children's Medicaid Demonstration, described in the next section. Established in May 1987, the program was intended to enroll up to 2,500 children with a large pediatric group called University Pediatric Associates (UPA) that would provide primary physician services and authorize all referral care. By November 1989, 1,166 children were enrolled. Plans were developed to offer a comparable program to adults—Physician Case Management Program 2 (PCMP 2)—beginning in late 1989. The UPA receives an actuarially determined capitation payment for primary care (Type 2, except that payment is made to the group as opposed to an individual

* New York State Department of Health, "Report to the Legislature on the Implementation of the Medicaid Reform Act of 1984," Bureau of Medical Care, Office of Health System Management, Albany, NY, 1990.

PCM) and has an opportunity to participate in savings in the referral account residuals. Only 80 percent of the capitation is initially available; the remaining 20 percent functions as a withhold. Early and periodic screening, diagnosis, and treatment (EPSDT) is paid FFS outside of the capitation at the request of federal authorities.

Although this is a small program, certain features of this model and its evaluation merit its inclusion in the universe of programs being studied. It is also the only New York State Medicaid primary care management program for which some cost and use data are available.

Research method

The quasi-experimental design evaluation of cost effectiveness performed for the waiver renewal process involved creating a comparison group of children living in Erie County who were in conventional FFS. This group was called the "universal set" and reflected the cost and use experience of the age strata that were used to set capitation rates in PCMP. The analysis examined persons who had at least six months' eligibility prior to enrollment to permit control for prior use—a common technique to try to eliminate differences associated with selection bias rather than program intervention effects. The levels of cost per person then were compared to the levels per person in the universal set for the same period to produce a prior use adjustment factor for each actuarial class.

This adjustment factor then was applied to the enrollment year results for both groups to produce an adjusted comparison (i.e., what the cost per person would have been if prior year differences not existed). The final adjustment was to produce an enrolled, population-blended rate that reflected the composition of the population in terms of a single measure. The same was done for the comparison group so that differences in actuarial classes could be aggregated to calculate overall savings.

The measures available for comparison were based on claims and capitation data and were all, of necessity, in dollar amounts (in a capitated program, no primary care claims or encounter forms are normally produced). The measures included referral account expenditures (inpatient, laboratory and x-ray, specialists, etc.); primary care expenditures; emergency department expenditures, and EPSDT expenditures (called the Child/Teen Health Program, or C/THP, in New York). Use was aggregated in the referral account because this account was used to determine whether savings were available to share with UPA. The period examined was May 1987 to February 1989.

Findings

With respect to selection bias, the PCMP enrollees in three of four actuarial classes had lower previous year use than universal set members, suggesting some evidence of favorable selection bias into the plan. The findings with respect to the referral account suggested it was 66 percent lower than for enrollees versus the comparison group ($6.50 versus $19.05). Unfortunately, lack of detail on the nature of the source of these savings makes it impossible to determine whether this result was caused primarily by inpatient use, which it might have been given the magnitude of reduction. On the other hand, the small number of admissions in this group could contribute to unreliable estimates.

Primary care expenditures were 38 percent higher in the same period for enrollees ($11.37 versus $8.22), suggesting that some offsetting of referral care might be occurring. Emergency department expenditures declined by 22 percent for enrollees. This finding is particularly interesting since after-hour coverage for this UPA group involved the referral of enrollees to Children's Hospital. Thus, there was no explicit gatekeeping of the emergency department in this program. Consequently, the reduction observed is almost certainly due to enrollee self-diversion to a PCP who was now required to be available at least during regular office hours. This particular finding has never been directly reported previously. The final finding indicated that C/THP expenditures were higher among enrollees than among nonenrollees in the universal set.

In summary, the overall cost saving associated with the PCMP-1 was a 32.8 percent lower rate of expenditures. Adding back the increases due to higher C/THP decreased the savings to 29.1 percent.

Assessment

The findings from this small voluntary program for children must be recognized as having limited generalizability. In addition, the use of dollars rather than direct-use measures confounds price- and volume-related changes. The lack of detail on changes in the component parts of the referral account is disappointing. Furthermore, to control for prior use, the study was restricted to persons who had two years of continuous eligibility. Finally, there are no statistical tests on differences; this omission is important since the group sizes are relatively small and dollar amounts are subject to large variations.

There are some strengths in this analysis, however. The model is straightforward and suitable for urban settings. A legitimate attempt has been made to control for selection bias using a variation of the prior-use technique. The finding on emergency department reductions—notwithstanding that the emergency department is used for after-hour coverage—is instructive regarding how the availability of a primary care manager induces voluntary diversion of care from the emergency department. As noted earlier, this is the only analysis available from New York State's multiple models that presents findings on cost effects after controlling for selection bias.

Children's Medicaid Program of Suffolk County (New York)

Information sources

This program assessment was based on the July 1989 final report on physician reimbursement and continuing care under Medicaid, prepared for the HCFA and the Hartford Foundation.*

Program description

From the report abstract: A demonstration to test the effects of case management on utilization and expenditures for children covered by Medicaid was conducted between July 1, 1983, and December 31, 1985, in Suffolk County, New York. Physicians and children eligible for AFDC in the demonstration areas were asked to enroll in the Children's Medicaid Program (CMP). The program was voluntary for both physicians and beneficiaries. Children who were enrolled in the program were guaranteed eligibility for a minimum of one year. Physicians were randomly assigned to one of two case management payment groups: (1) a capitation group that received fixed monthly payments for all primary care and that was at risk for the cost of referred services and (2) an FFS group that received higher visit fees than under the regular Medicaid program but was not at financial risk for referred services. Approximately 80 physicians and 4,000 children were enrolled in the program during its 2½-year life. The program was funded jointly by the John A. Hartford Foundation of New York and HCFA.

Benefits derived from the CMP included (1) its acceptability to PCPs (as evidenced by high rates of participation and satisfaction), (2) its ability to increase patient access to PCPs (as reflected by higher physician visit rates and greater compliance with medical standards for minimum visit rates for younger children), and (3) higher Medicaid beneficiary satisfaction with the care received under the CMP.

Research method

This study used a quasi-experimental design with a before and after comparison group. Two experimental groups were used: (1) a capitation group and (2) an FFS group. Two comparison groups also were used: (1) a group that was in the same geographic area but was recertified for AFDC either one month prior to or one month after the demonstration group and (2) an out-of-area (but still in the same

---

* S. Davidson, G. Fleming, M. Hohlen, L. Manheim, B. Shapiro, and S. Wermer, "Physician Reimbursement and Continuing Care Under Medicaid" (final report prepared for HCFA and the John A. Hartford Foundation, Grant Nos. 11-P-98052 [HCFA] and 83185-3H [Hartford], July 1989). *See also* M. Hohlen, L. Manheim, G. Fleming, S. Davidson, B. Yudkowsky, S. Wermer, and G. Wheatley, "Access to Office-Based Physicians Under Capitation Reimbursement and Medicaid Case Management: Findings from the Children's Medicaid Program," *Medical Care* 28, no. 1 (1990): 59–68.

city) group that was being recertified for AFDC. The in-area group was used to estimate utilization and expenditures that would have occurred in the absence of the CMP. As described above, physicians, not beneficiaries, were randomly assigned a payment method. Participation in the program was voluntary and enrollees were free to choose their own PCM.

Baseline claims data were used to measure prior utilization and demographic variables. Utilization variables measured included PCP visits, specialist visits, clinic and outpatient visits, emergency department services, inpatient admissions, and inpatient LOS. Cost data also were collected for these variables as well as for dental, pharmacy, freestanding laboratory work, clinical psychology, and other services. Because the capitated group filed encounter forms rather than claims, underreporting for this group was audited via medical records review. Utilization was found to be underestimated for this group by about 10 percent.

Ordinary least squares and logit regression were used in the analysis. Age, gender, race, month enrolled, and group membership were used as covariates in the analysis.

Findings

The possibility of selection bias is present in this study for at least two reasons: (1) the program was voluntary, thus introducing differences between participants and nonparticipants; and (2) participants were guaranteed eligibility throughout the demonstration, regardless of their change in status. Selection bias was analyzed. Those who refused to enter the demonstration had higher baseline hospital costs. The augmented FFS group had higher hospital costs than the in-area comparison group, while the capitated group had lower hospital costs than the in-area comparison group at baseline. Differences also were found between the recertified group and the nonrecertified groups.

Utilization effects were reported relative to the in-area comparison group. The capitated group was not statistically significantly different from the in-area comparison group in terms of all physician visits but had a higher number of PCP visits and a lower number of specialist visits. Logit regression was performed to compare the probability of being hospitalized between the capitated group and the in-area comparison group and between the capitated group and the augmented FFS group. The capitated group was not statistically significantly different from the in-area comparison group, but members of this group were hospitalized significantly less often than were members of the augmented FFS group. The odds of being hospitalized for the capitated group were 77.5 percent of the odds of being hospitalized for the FFS group during the demonstration. However, these same differences were noted between the groups prior to the demonstration. No significant differences were seen in terms of emergency department visits between the capitated group and the in-area comparison group. Lower numbers of clinic visits were found for this group in relationship to the in-area comparison group.

In comparison to the in-area group, the augmented FFS group had higher overall physician visits and higher PCP visits. However, there was no significant difference between these groups in terms of specialist visits, emergency department visits, and hospital days. Lower numbers of clinic visits were seen relative to the in-area comparison group.

Cost findings also were reported relative to the in-area comparison group. Higher costs were reported for both groups for overall physician visits and PCP visits. Lower costs for clinic expenditures were seen for both groups. The capitated group had lower costs for specialist care, while no significant differences were seen between costs for the FFS group and the comparison group. Hospital expenditures were lower for the capitated group, while no significant difference was found between the FFS and the in-area comparison group. Although no significant differences were seen between the experimental groups and the in-area comparison group in terms of emergency department expenditures, the capitated group had lower costs due to the ability to recoup payments made without prior authorization.

Assessment

This study was extremely well designed but exhibits the problems with control relevant to a voluntary program. Because of the study's inability to randomly assign enrollees to the two experimental groups, as well as the voluntary nature of the program, the comparison groups were not equivalent at baseline. Therefore, differences in utilization between the two experimental groups and the comparison groups might have occurred in part because of selection rather than solely because of program effects, as noted in the HCFA report. The analysis is exceedingly well done, showing contrasts with several different subgroups in addition to the comparison between the experimental and study comparison groups. Contrasts with prior use also are available since eligibility histories are available for both experimental and comparison groups.

A major weakness of the study is that both case management models had a substantial increase in reimbursement as an incentive for physician participation. Therefore, there was no strict control group. Another problem exists in that physician participants were recruited from those who expressed an interest in the program. In addition, not all patients in a physician's practice were participants in the study. Thus, if the physician treated all Medicaid patients in the same way, the treatment effect might have been diluted.

As mentioned above, not all the groups were equivalent at baseline. In addition to the utilization differences noted above, the groups were different in terms of age and race. The recertified groups were different from the participants who volunteered or who were chosen from physician lists.

The primary limitation of the study is its lack of generalizability since it was restricted to AFDC children and not opened to all Medicaid beneficiaries. Another limitation lies in the urban nature of the program. If this type of program were to be implemented in a rural area where physicians rarely have practices that consist exclusively of Medicaid enrollees, the results might be significantly different.

Dayton (Ohio) Area Health Plan

Information sources

The principal source of data for this overview is the 1991 waiver renewal assessment, including the external evaluation of cost and use effects performed by RTI.*

Program description

Ohio has had a longstanding voluntary HMO enrollment program that has been widely available throughout the state, most notably in several major metropolitan areas. In 1987 planning began to introduce a mandatory HMO enrollment program (Type 3) in the Dayton area (Montgomery County), which at that time had a voluntary HMO enrollment of nearly 40 percent. The original plan was to establish an HIO that would contract with the state and in turn subcontract with participating HMOs. Several obstacles that arose to this arrangement included federal legislation that rendered it infeasible.

However, a local coordinating group, the Dayton Area Health Plan (DAHP), emerged as a de facto HIO, became the on-site intermediary, and developed the program in cooperation with the state. In addition to contracting with two preexisting IPA-model HMOs, DAHP established a third HMO—the Health Plan Network. This IPA-network HMO was designed to enroll all beneficiaries who did not choose one of the other two plans and also to act as an umbrella plan to allow other providers in the community not affiliated with these two HMOs to participate in the plan. There is a high degree of participation among providers in the community and a variety of methods for paying physicians, health centers, and hospitals among the three HMOs.

The program was made mandatory in 1989 for AFDC beneficiaries, and the phased-in implementation was begun for new eligibles. Other beneficiaries as yet unenrolled in an HMO converted at the time of recertification. Virtually full enrollment was achieved in the spring of 1990. As a mandatory program it is not susceptible to selection bias, although the phase-in plan probably ensured that enrollment among plans is not random. Total enrollment is approximately 40,000 with two plans having the preponderance of enrollees. There has been some resistance in the community to the program, and a lawsuit was filed by the local Legal Aid Society. Nevertheless, the state was able to negotiate an interim agreement to proceed with implementation.

Research method

The original evaluation design was intended to conduct a before and after analysis with person-level claims files for samples of beneficiaries from Dayton and from

---

* Research Triangle Institute, "Analyses of Medicaid Cost and Utilization Experience for Montgomery County Medicaid Recipients Under Mandatory HMO Enrollment" (prepared for the Ohio Department of Human Services, Division of Medical Assistance, under Contract No. 91-118AP, 1991).

Summit County (Akron), an appropriate comparison county without any Medicaid HMO enrollment. Encounter data were acquired directly from HMOs, which were required only to submit aggregate monthly reports of utilization. Due to a serious data problem in the historical eligibility files in Ohio's MMIS, it was not possible to conduct the study entirely as planned. An alternative strategy was adopted to do a cross-sectional, post-year-only comparison for the ten-month period from July 1989 to April 1990, the first period after implementation that was not contaminated by the state's data file problem.

The evaluation focused on several measures of use, including the two-part model for physician, emergency department, ancillary, prescription, and inpatient use. The prescription data were deemed unreliable. Some underreporting was noted in one of the three plans (an interplan comparison was also done but is not reported here). The cost-effectiveness measures included capitation payments in Dayton, FFS payments in Summit, and two estimates of expected FFS equivalent expenditures for Dayton-area beneficiaries. Statistical tests were performed in multivariate models of utilization that controlled for individual person differences in age, gender, race, and duration of eligibility, with separate analyses for adults and children.

Findings

The overall findings reported indicated that there were relatively few significant differences between the two counties after controlling for demographic differences. For example, there was a higher rate of inpatient use in the unadjusted findings for Dayton, but this higher rate resulted from higher levels of delivery-related stays and from a higher proportion of women of childbearing age as compared to Summit. That inpatient use was not lower in the HMOs in Dayton was somewhat surprising, but the inpatient use rate for that county is among the highest in the state. In addition, with 40 percent of beneficiaries already enrolled in HMOs in the premandatory period, the HMO effect was perhaps diluted.

Notwithstanding some evidence of underreporting in Dayton, there were virtually no differences in physician service or ancillary use between the two counties. There was evidence of about a 20 percent reduction in the probability of an emergency department visit in Dayton versus the comparison county. Closer examination of this difference suggested substantial interplan variation in the rigor of their gatekeeping.

Cost savings accrued to the state by definition since the capitation rates were set on a discount from expected FFS expenditures. The analysis attempted to estimate more precisely whether the contractual savings were associated with reductions in resources consumed by beneficiaries based on FFS equivalent costs or on imputed prices for rendered services. One approach was to use HMO encounter data to estimate the volume of services and then to impute Medicaid prices to these services to arrive at FFS equivalent service expenditures. Underreporting in service volumes and problems in price imputation prevented this estimate from being reliable. The second approach was to estimate the FFS experience expected for Dayton beneficiaries by applying the FFS experience of Summit County beneficiaries through a statistical technique called means replacement. This estimation approach indicated that the capitation payment was about 10 percent less than the expected level of expenditure.

Assessment

As with the Wisconsin HMO program, the mandatory enrollment in HMOs in Montgomery County, Ohio, was implemented relatively quickly and generally successfully with a high level of provider participation. The evidence suggests that modest savings are being achieved with levels of use that are quite comparable with those for the FFS conventional program. Unfortunately, the evaluation planned for this site, which would have been perhaps the most detailed picture of a mandatory HMO enrollment program, especially in terms of utilization, had to be drastically modified. Ironically, the modification in Ohio was required not because of missing encounter data from prepaid providers or plans but because of problems in the state's Medicaid eligibility history files.

Oregon Medicaid Physician Care Organization Program

Information sources

The sources for this description were the state's waiver application, including a cost-effectiveness study performed by Coopers & Lybrand and a review of the program included in a paper by W. Pete Welch entitled "Giving Physicians Incentives to Contain Costs under Medicare: Lessons from Medicaid."* Welch's work relied on state waiver applications and other state-provided information.

Program description

Oregon obtained waivers in 1984 to introduce a capitated primary care management program in the principal urban areas of the state, with the ultimate aim of taking the program statewide if successful. The program required mandatory enrollment of AFDC beneficiaries in the operational counties with approved physician care organizations or HMOs. By June 1989, 53,000 enrollees in nine counties had enrolled with one of fifteen primary care organizations and one HMO. The primary care organizations typically are physician groups that can assume responsibility for directly providing a wide range of primary and ancillary services in return for a capitation payment. The capitation is based on 100 percent of the expected FFS as determined from the experience of the nonenrolled population and adjusted for county cost-of-living differences.

---

* Coopers & Lybrand, "Cost Effectiveness for the PCO/HMO Program for the Period March 1985 through September 1988" (prepared for the Department of Human Services, State of Oregon, 1989); W. P. Welch, "Giving Physicians Incentives to Contain Costs Under Medicaid," *Health Care Financing Review* 12, no. 2 (1990): 103–12.

The primary care organization is also responsible for authorizing remaining care, including outpatient, drug, and inpatient use that are paid by the state, with the primary care organization able to participate in residuals in these accounts due to lower-than-expected use. There is a ceiling of $3.25 of savings per enrollee per month for the primary care organization. Thus, the primary care organization, which is expected to assign each individual to a PCP, is functioning like a Type 2 program, although it is not typically the case that the individual primary care manager is at direct financial risk. In the HMO (Kaiser Permanente), the capitation rate is paid for the full scope of covered services, and no direct incentive payments are available to the HMO. We have excluded the HMO from this discussion since it is not explicitly treated in the waiver application.

The program ultimately is targeted to be implemented statewide, with its mandatory status conditional on sufficient provider participation. Plans exist to employ competitive bidding more extensively. Also built into the program design is a plan to extend the coverage to nearly all noninstitutionalized Medicaid beneficiaries.

Research method

The principal analysis available is the Coopers & Lybrand study, which focused primarily on actual capitation plus noncapitated expenditures for primary care organization enrollees versus average FFS experience for nonenrollees. An adjustment was made for county-level differences but not for potential differences in personal characteristics of enrollees versus nonenrollees. Despite this program being mandatory, there might have been important population-based differences between urban versus non-urban dwellers that affected patterns of use and cost. Also, no attention was paid to the HMO-enrolling group insofar as they might have been different from primary care organization enrollees. Their omission might have had a bearing on the findings.

The analysis examined expenditure experience in total and by inpatient, outpatient, pharmacy, and physician service expenditures for the four years 1985–1988. Unfortunately, as noted by Welch, the final year (1987–1988) showed an enormous increase in savings that very possibly resulted from unreported claims at the time analysis was done. Coopers & Lybrand did an incurred-but-not-reported estimate but acknowledged that it might have understated actual experience. For this reason, using the prior year probably would yield a more reliable estimate of savings.

The analysis was done county by county, with the Portland area counties grouped as the tri-county area. Because the program began there, it provides the most complete program effect picture. As noted above, the measures used were expenditures rather than visits, claims, encounters, procedures, etc. Therefore, there is no way to ascertain patterns of use independent of payment. An extensive quality-of-care evaluation was done by the professional review organization (PRO), but relatively small sample sizes do not permit this evaluation to inform effects on use. In addition, the analysis excludes maternity care because the intervention is not expected to affect use and cost experience in this area; consequently, the incentives are not applied to maternity care.

Findings

The annual aggregate savings per enrollee per month were a loss of $1.79 in 1985 and savings of $2.98 and $3.36 in 1986 and 1987. The 1988 savings were reported as $9.91 but (for reasons noted above) this finding is suspect. Extrapolating the 1987 savings to 53,000 enrollees would suggest annual savings of approximately $2.0 million, net of reported administrative costs.

With respect to service categories, we again refer to the 1987 experience. Physician service expenditures (including services paid by FFS outside of the capitation rate) were 19 percent higher in the tri-county area, with smaller increases noted in the other counties. Much of this difference was due to the shifting of care from outpatient to physician services as outpatient expenditures dropped by nearly 80 percent in the tri-counties but by less than half of that amount in the other counties. This suggests that while some of the reduction could be attributed to lower emergency department use (not measured separately), it could also have been caused by a shifting of primary care and ancillary use away from outpatient departments.

Prescription expenditures present a mixed picture with relatively small increases and reductions noted for PCO enrollees, varying by county. For example, there was an increase of 6 percent in the tri-county area and 4 percent in Marion and Polk Counties but a reduction of 8 percent in Lane County. The major reduction in expenditures (and presumably in use, since DRG payment methods were the same for primary care organization and non–primary care organization enrollees) was in the inpatient realm. Inpatient expenditures dropped 31 percent, 41 percent, and 23 percent in the three county areas noted above. This drop resulted in substantial incentive payments being available in all the counties and for virtually all the primary care organizations.

Assessment

The analysis relied on here has many limitations in method, design, data, and indicators in terms of its usefulness to rigorously evaluate the effects of the primary care organization program. At best, it is simply an attempt to estimate what cost savings might be associated with the introduction of the program. Despite these limitations, it does present a reasonably strong case for what are apparently substantial reductions in inpatient expenditures, which are compatible with the incentive payment system being employed. Since the contracting with the primary care organizations creates reasonably large groups of enrollees for risk-pooling purposes (with stop-loss coverage also available), individual PCCM has been integrated into a model that also accommodates inpatient cost risk-sharing. The lack of detail on individual plans prevents any assessment of how risk is shared with or transmitted to individual physicians. One would also be interested in knowing what types of inpatient utilization review practices have been adopted to achieve these impressive results.

As noted earlier, the findings with respect to use are based on expenditures. This choice leaves opaque many of the dynamics of primary care organization–style PCCM. Particularly interesting would be determining whether emergency department use declined or whether the outpatient reductions have resulted largely from the shifting of primary care and ancillary use from outpatient departments to doctors' offices. Finally, the findings are now three years old. Since the expansion of the program has continued, it would be noteworthy to assess whether continued inpatient use reductions are occurring. In addition, as Welch notes, the reliability of the population base not enrolled in a primary care organization and its FFS experience will diminish as the program expands. It is not clear, therefore, how future rates will be computed for both payment and evaluation purposes.

HealthPASS of Philadelphia (Pennsylvania)

Information sources

The study source was an external evaluation dated August 1989 prepared by the SOLON Consulting Group, Ltd., in conjunction with the Center for Demographic Studies, Duke University, for the Pennsylvania Department of Public Welfare (DPW).* It covered the period between January 1, 1987, and August 31, 1988. The purpose of the evaluation was to meet HCFA requirements for the continuation of waivers for the HealthPASS program. A supplemental evaluation, dated January 1990, was also performed by the Solon Consulting Group.† This assessment examines first the original evaluation, then the supplement.

Program description

HealthPASS is an HIO responsible for providing acute care to Medical Assistance (MA) beneficiaries in five districts in south and west Philadelphia. At the initiation of the HealthPASS program, this area contained 28 percent (102,000 enrollees) of Philadelphia's MA population, which enabled the enrollment of the targeted number of 100,000 beneficiaries recommended by the task force. At the time of the evaluation, 87,000 beneficiaries were enrolled. This geographic area also contained approximately half of the MA providers in Philadelphia County. In addition to HealthPASS, two HMOs with the combined maximum capacity to serve 5,000 Medicaid recipients provided services to over 2,000 MA enrollees.

HealthPASS is a Type 2 program, an HIO in which PCPs, physician groups, or community health centers serve as case managers. Within certain guidelines, enrollees can change case managers at any time. Case managers receive a capitated payment, adjusted for age, gender, and MA category, for each enrollee and are responsible for locating, coordinating, and monitoring all primary care and other

---

* SOLON Consulting Group, Ltd., and the Center for Demographic Studies, Duke University, "HealthPASS External Evaluation" (prepared under contract to the Pennsylvania Department of Public Welfare, Harrisburg, PA, 1989).

† SOLON Consulting Group, Ltd., and the Center for Demographic Studies, Duke University, "HealthPASS External Evaluation: Final Report Supplement" (prepared under contract to the Pennsylvania Department of Public Welfare, Harrisburg, PA, 1990).

medical services for recipients. Authorization must be obtained for most covered services with the exception of emergency services, emergency ambulance transportation, family planning, eyeglasses, and dental services. Primary care managers are at risk for all physician services and outpatient laboratory and x-ray services. Half the capitation rate is paid at the beginning of each month, and half is held for the payment of referral services, outpatient laboratory fees, and x-rays. The PCP receives any surplus that exists at the end of the year. Deficits are charged against future capitation (up to 20 percent per month) with a stop-loss arrangement to insure against large losses for referrals. Each PCP has responsibility for a hospitalization management reserve fund that covers inpatient services, emergency department charges, ambulance fees, and home health services. The fund is created by the allocation of a capitated amount per recipient. Primary care physicians are paid a bonus if savings from reduced rates of hospitalization accrue at the end of the contract year. However, all PCPs are denied a bonus from the hospitalization fund if the aggregate hospital fund is depleted.

The comparison of cost between groups is confounded by the fact that traditional Medicaid in Pennsylvania uses its own DRG prices while the HIO pays capitated rates per hospital day.

Research methods for the initial evaluation

The target group included most categorically eligible and medically needy MA recipients except for those in the following categories: those already enrolled in HMOs, residents of nursing homes and intermediate care facilities for the mentally retarded, those eligible through monthly spend-downs, H-grant recipients, and state blind pension recipients.

A cross-sectional design was used to examine the effects of the program. A comparison group, based on geography, was composed of those in the FFS system in the rest of the city. Evaluators compared rates (adjusted for gender, age, and race but not for case mix) for the various utilization variables. Two years of data were given for most of the variables of interest. However, no before and after analyses were done.

Utilization variables included were hospital admissions (measured by hospital bills), hospital outpatient department visits, physician visits, and emergency department visits. Cost was measured in terms of total cost as the product of price per service times the quantity of services purchased. Data sources included claims data for the comparison group and encounter data for the HealthPASS group.

Findings

Utilization. Service use was examined, adjusting for age, gender, and race. Race categories were white, black, and "other." "Other" consisted mostly of Hispanic for the non-HIO group and Asian for the HIO group. Comparisons between the HIO and non-HIO groups were made. Hospital use under the HIO was less than that of the non-HIO group with reductions generally being larger for persons in the middle age ranges over all groups. Hospital use was much lower for black males under the HIO than for black males in the non-HIO group. Outpatient visits also were lower for the HIO groups relative to the non-HIO groups. In 1987, it appears that some site shifting might have caused inpatient service reduction, with outpatient care being substituted for inpatient care more for whites and not as much for the other groups. Blacks in 1987 had generally lower outpatient than inpatient utilization. For the "other" group, lower outpatient use was also clearly evident. However, in 1988, outpatient visits were almost always lower for all six groups under the HIO. Competing interpretations were suggested for this reduction. The first was that it could reflect a real change in practice patterns; the second was that it could reflect a change in name. That is, a visit labeled outpatient in 1987 might have been labeled a physician visit in 1988. Whatever the explanation, it appears that the HIO was not substituting outpatient for inpatient care.

It appears that the HIO increased access to physician services for most of the groups. Again, this might have been the result of a change in the label given to the service (i.e., outpatient care by another name). However, the "other" group had lower numbers of physician visits under the HIO in comparison to the non-HIO group. Reduced access to hospital and outpatient services was also seen for this group. Since this group was primarily Asian, language and cultural barriers to access might also have been important.

Last, in comparison to the non-HIO group, the HIO appeared to strikingly reduce the inappropriate use of emergency department services. In addition, in comparison to 1987, the 1988 emergency department use by the non-HIO group was lower.

Cost. HealthPASS guarantees an initial savings of 10 percent of the FFS costs of the MA program for the population served. In this type of program, the HIO is put at financial risk for all specified services to HealthPASS enrollees. After the first year of operation, Penn Health reported a pretax loss of $7.8 million. It was determined that the initial capitation rate was set too low, at an effective rate of 80 percent rather than the agreed on 90 percent of the FFS adjusted average per capita cost. The risk-sharing agreement was altered and a $2 million loss limit was set for the first two years.

Costs were analyzed by summing all payments to all providers and dividing by all eligibles for the same time period. The sum of the provider payments by provider type and in total was divided by the total number of eligible persons to obtain a cost per person per year rate. Costs were then compared to the same rate for the traditional MA program. The analyses suggest that HealthPASS is effective in controlling utilization but not the price per unit. On the other hand, the traditional MA program is effective in controlling price but not as effective as HealthPASS in controlling utilization. For example, the HIO was able to reduce inpatient utilization but was not as effective at reducing cost in comparison to the non-HIO group since the non-HIO group paid a DRG rate for hospital inpatient care and the HIO did not have authority to use an inpatient hospital payment alternative.

Overall, the cost results were mixed. Females, particularly those of childbearing age, were less profitable for the HIO than males. Age differences were observed as well, as HealthPASS seems to have spent less on the elderly than did the traditional MA. However, this might also have been a function of excluded long-term care services. By specific service, HIO payments for inpatient services were generally lower than traditional MA for males, but not for females. Similar results were observed for outpatient services. However, higher payments for whites under the HIO were seen in comparison to the other two groups, all relative to traditional MA. In the category of physician services, the HIO had higher costs over all subgroups. Last, strikingly lower costs were observed for emergency department services under the HIO relative to the non-HIO groups over all population subgroups.

Research methods for the supplemental evaluation

A second analysis was undertaken to adjust for two concerns in the initial analysis: (1) case-mix differences between the groups and (2) differences in exposure time for the two groups. This analysis focused on specific subgroups within the HIO's catchment area: (1) females with obstetric and gynecological problems, (2) persons with drug or alcohol problems, (3) persons with mental health diagnoses, (4) persons over 65 years of age, (5) infants, and (6) all others. The GOM case-mix methodology* was used to make case-mix adjustments in the analyses. Additional analyses were conducted for those with cancer, hypertension, and diabetes. Data used in the analysis were DPW recipient data, DPW Medicaid paid claims for Philadelphia County, encounter claims from HealthPASS, and mortality data from the Pennsylvania Department of Health Vital Statistics Record system. Lifetable analysis, which includes time in the sense of duration, was used to address the relationship between periods of eligibility and service use.

Findings

The GOM analysis distinguished case-mix groups for each of the subpopulations described above. Four types or groups were found for the drug and alcohol subpopulation. Median length of hospital stay was found to be similar between the HIO and non-HIO comparison groups, both in general and by case mix group. The pattern of LOS and probability of admission differed between the case-mix groups, but the pattern between HIO and non-HIO groups was fairly consistent. No statistically significant differences were detected between the two groups for either hospital or community mortality. Hospital costs were lower for the HIO for this entire subpopulation but higher for two of the case mix types. However, overall hospital costs were lower because of the lower probability of admission under the HIO. The HIO also spent more on average per day for community care than did the FFS sector.

Four types were found for the mental health subpopulation. Again, although differences were found between the types, the pattern of service use was found to be consistent between the HIO and the FFS sector. Both hospital and community

---

* M. A. Woodbury and K. G. Manton, "A New Procedure for Analysis of Medical Classification," *Methods of Information in Medicine* 21 (1982): 210–20.

mortality rates were lower under the HIO. Hospital admissions were reduced by 1 percent under the HIO, and hospitals were paid less for this service. Hospital costs were found to be generally lower under the HIO. However, the HIO spent more for children than did the FFS sector. Community costs were higher under the HIO for this subpopulation, implying a substitution of this type of care for hospital care. Since the system paid more for community care and less for hospital care than the FFS sector, the HIO essentially broke even for this subpopulation.

Four types were also used to analyze the obstetric-gynecology subpopulation. Again, the case-mix groups consistently received services differentially in the HIO and FFS sectors. In a comparison of median LOS in the community, the analysis found the probability of admission for the HIO group to be slightly less than for the non-HIO group, but the HIO tended to admit people sooner than the FFS sector. Mortality under the HIO was found to be higher, and hospital mortality was statistically significantly higher. Hospital admissions were 7 percent lower for the HIO than for the FFS sector. Thus, the HIO controlled costs by spending less per day on hospital care. For all but the acutely ill group, community services substituted for hospital services for the HIO group. Thus, higher community care costs were seen under the HIO, but the reduction in hospital use more than offset the higher cost of community services.

Four pure types were used to define the newborn subpopulation—all those less than one year old. Again, differential patterns of service existed over the four types with consistent patterns seen between the HIO and FFS sectors. The same control over admissions was seen in this subpopulation as in the others, with admission probabilities being lower under the HIO except for all but the very sick infants. Hospital costs were only slightly lower for the HIO while its medical services costs were higher.

Three pure types characterized the over-65 subpopulation. Once again, the patterns of service use were similar for the case-mix groups, with the HIO and FFS systems performing similarly. However, the HIO did not control hospital admissions as well for this subpopulation as it did for the others. The older age group was much more likely to be hospitalized under the HIO than under FFS. Hospitalization under the HIO occurred sooner as well as more often. Mortality in the hospital and in the community was lower under the HIO. Although admissions were higher, the HIO had lower costs for hospital care for all the case-mix groups (noting here that most hospital care for the over-65 age group was paid for by Medicare). As before, higher costs per day were observed for community care for the HIO than for the FFS sector, although the difference here was small.

The "other" subpopulation included all those who did not fall into any of the above subpopulations. Four pure types were used, although fewer pure types were indicated in the analysis. Again, LOS by case-mix group was consistent between the HIO and the FFS sectors. The HIO controlled hospital admissions selectively across the case-mix groups. Hospital mortality was higher for the HIO than for the FFS system, while no differences were seen between the groups in terms of community mortality. Hospital costs per day of exposure were lower for the HIO for two of the case-mix groups but higher for the other two. Community costs were higher per day for the HIO.

Assessment

The comparability of the groups was questionable in the initial analysis since differences in the medical conditions between the two groups were not controlled for in the analysis. The mortality analysis showed that the HIO group almost always had lower mortality rates than the non-HIO group. The most likely explanation for this finding is that there were case-mix differences between the groups, rather than that the HIO actually reduced mortality for most of the subgroups examined in the analysis. Another reason to suspect their generalizability is in the racial composition of the two groups. The ''other'' categories were primarily Hispanic in the non-HIO group, while the HIO group ''other'' category was primarily Asian. Thus, although the use of a geographic comparison group might have been appropriate, the selection of such a group should more carefully address similarities of the geographic areas to be compared.

Although the GOM analysis provided findings for case-mix groups, severity of illness within the disease categories was not controlled for in the analysis.

The potential for selection bias due to HealthPASS eligibles voluntarily enrolling in an HMO was not explored but did not contaminate the results of the analysis as performed here.

The major weaknesses of this evaluation are its methods and choice of variables. In the first analysis, the comparisons were rather gross, with no tests of statistical significance of differences between the two groups. The second analysis used a method known and understood by relatively few, thus hindering the usefulness of the findings. The choice of variables in the second analysis, where outpatient and physician visits were grouped together, obscures comparison between the two analyses and is not as useful to the consumer of this information as two separate variables would be. Last, the major contribution of this study is that it offers an example of how such programs might function in a large, urban setting.

Utah's Choice of Health Care Delivery Programs

Information sources

The principal sources of information included the state's waiver application cost-effectiveness study done by Peat Marwick.* More detailed, though earlier, data are available from the MPE and the in-depth study conducted in Utah and published by Long and Settle.†

---

* KPMG Peat Marwick, ''Waiver Continuation Request for the State of Utah'' (prepared for the Division of Health Care Financing, Utah Department of Health, Salt Lake City, UT, 1989).

† Office of Research and Demonstrations (ORD), *Medicaid Program Evaluation: Final Report*, Report No. MPE 9.2, eds. J. Holahan, J. Bell, and G. S. Adler (Baltimore, MD: Health Care Financing Administration, 1987); S. Long and R. Settle, ''An Evaluation of Utah Primary Care Case Management Program for Medicaid Recipients,'' *Medical Care* 26, no. 11 (1988): 102–32.

Program description

The Utah program was implemented in March 1982 as a mandatory enrollment program for beneficiaries in the state's most populous counties (the Salt Lake City area has 75 percent of all eligibles). The program was designed to enable beneficiaries either to select a primary care gatekeeper or to join participating HMOs. HMO participation has been limited and has been a viable option only in the Salt Lake City area. Of 59,000 eligible persons, approximately 14,000 are in HMOs and 25,000 are enrolled with PCCMs, with the remainder in traditional Medicaid in areas where the program was not available (as of June 1987). Limited findings are available on the experience of HMO enrollees, so this discussion focuses on primary care gatekeeper enrollees only.

Primary care physicians and organizations may qualify to become primary care case managers and are paid FFS with neither incentives nor a case management fee (Type 1). The state has expressed an interest in instituting a case management fee, capitation, or both for primary care managers at some time in the future. The program is targeted toward all eligible groups. The primary care manager is expected to provide primary care directly and to authorize referral care, but has no financial incentives. Given the concentration of the eligible population in the Salt Lake City area, the findings reported pertain primarily to an urban-based intervention. However, since HMO enrollment also took place predominantly in that area as well, it is not clear how differential enrollment patterns might affect observed program impacts.

Research methods

The Utah experience illustrates rather vividly the potential for discrepancies in asserted savings and effects depending on either source of assertions, quality of data and analysis, or timing of the analysis. The state's waiver applications and the most recent external assessment suggest modest though substantial savings. The basic approach employed is to compare adjusted expenditure per HMO and primary care gatekeeper enrollees to the mean expenditures for non-case-managed enrollees. The adjustment pertained primarily to developing a weighting factor for each of the various eligible groups as represented in the enrolled versus nonenrolled populations. No other adjustments were made, so individual differences between enrollees and nonenrollees were not controlled for or ruled out regarding their contribution to savings. Administrative costs were accounted for in the asserted savings.

A rigorous evaluation of the early experience (1983–1984) performed by Long and Settle was at sharp variance with the state's appraisals at that time. In the analysis they did, complex samples of enrollees and not-yet-enrollees were drawn, and their prior levels of use were calculated to control for selection bias or differential or nonrandom rates of enrollment. In addition, their models of use controlled for other effects that might have been expected to influence levels of use including age, gender, race, and county of residence.

The source of their data was claims, which they structured into encounter data with which they could conduct a relatively sophisticated assessment of some of the dynamics of PCCM. The variables used included physician visits to primary care and specialty care doctors, emergency department and hospital outpatient clinic visits (not separated), prescriptions, and clinic visits. They did not examine inpatient use since they used a brief interval of eligibility to examine ambulatory effects. They also employed the two-part model of probability of use and use-for-users to explore gatekeeper effects in the multivariate analyses. The approach is one of the most extensive analyses done to date on a gatekeeper program, although it came very early in the program's implementation.

Findings

The June 1988 cost-effectiveness study suggested that 1987 savings were 17.0 percent for HMO enrollees and 8.9 percent for primary care gatekeeper enrollees. These savings were approximately twice as high as those noted in 1986 (7.2 percent and 4.2 percent, respectively), suggesting that cumulative increases in program effects might be occurring. Although the Peat Marwick study presented only expenditure data, it is possible to see what service types contributed to differences in terms of inpatient, physician and ancillary, outpatient, and pharmacy costs. For the AFDC categorically eligible population, inpatient expenditures in the PCCM program were 8.2 percent lower than for the traditional FFS population, while outpatient expenditures were 11.9 percent lower. It is not possible, however, to determine how much of this was emergency department reduction and how much was outpatient care shifted to primary care gatekeepers. Physician and laboratory and x-ray expenditures (combined) were 13 percent higher in the gatekeeper population than in the non–primary care managed group. Pharmacy service expenditures were slightly (4 percent) lower in the gatekeeper group.

While conducting the analysis using the two-part model, Long and Settle presented an aggregate estimate of program effects on ambulatory use. Primary care visits increased by 30 percent, and specialist visits went up by 12 percent. Prescriptions also increased by over 40 percent with the only reduction in ambulatory use being an 11.5 percent drop in emergency department and outpatient department use. The authors suggested these findings were due to emergency department use but could not disentangle these differences.

Insofar as the two-part model is concerned, Long and Settle made an important observation. They noted that most of the increases were due to substantial increases in the probability of a visit, while the use-for-users was largely unchanged. The implication of this, they suggested, was that the gatekeeper intervention had a significant access-enhancing effect, particularly for those persons who (prior to implementation) might not have had a relationship with a PCP. They further argued that there was a complementary relationship between primary care, specialty care, and prescription use, rather than a substitution effect, with this particular population. It should be recalled that there were no incentives to primary care gatekeepers to avoid making referrals.

While acknowledging that these findings pertain to an early period of implementation and might well change over time, Long and Settle saw no evidence of savings associated with the program. They did not examine costs directly, however. They noted that overall there was a 25 percent increase in ambulatory use, which represented about 55 percent of beneficiary expenditures. Though inpatient use was not examined, the evaluators implied that the gatekeeper approach was unlikely to make substantial differences in this type of use.

Assessment

As suggested in the methods section, the waiver-related documentation is relatively weak in its credibility regarding actual program effects and savings. However, it does build on several years of sustained operating experience, which of itself is a useful contribution. On the other hand, the omission of a detailed study of HMO enrollees prevents drawing a conclusive picture regarding the impact of gatekeeper enrollment. One also has to question the true comparability of the nonenrolled population inasmuch as they come from a substantially less urban population and probably differ on several other characteristics.

Long and Settle's assessment is a methodologically impressive one that provides a richly detailed picture of the dynamics of gatekeeping and, in their findings, of the lack of substitution of primary care for specialty care. It must be emphasized that the data used in this study are from 1983 and 1984, in the early period of implementation. It is possible, if not probable, that stronger program effects might be detectable now. The Peat Marwick study, though dramatically different in its analytical approach, methodological rigor, and reliability, does provide some indication that program effects might accumulate over time (1987 savings were larger than those for 1986). In particular, it is unlikely that initial improvement in access is as prominent as it originally was. Whether that means that increases in use previously observed are still as dramatic or even evident is unknown.

Kitsap (Washington) Sound Care Plan

Information sources

The two principal sources for information on this program were an evaluation performed by the Health Policy Analysis program at the University of Washington dated July 24, 1989, and a report on the structural and incentive features of the program contained in "Giving Physicians Incentives to Contain Costs under Medicare: Lessons from Medicaid"—an Urban Institute working paper by W. Pete Welch.*

Program description

The Kitsap Sound Care Plan is a PCCM program operated by Kitsap Physician Services (KPS) as an HIO under contract to the State of Washington Medicaid

* University of Washington, "Evaluation of the Kitsap Sound Care Plan: Access, Quality, and Cost-Effectiveness" (Seattle, WA: Department of Health Services, 1989); W. P. Welch, "Giving Physicians Incentives to Contain Costs Under Medicaid," *Health Care Financing Review* 12, no. 2 (1990): 103–12.

program. This mandatory program was initiated in February 1986 in two small counties, Kitsap and Mason. There are currently approximately 6,500 AFDC beneficiaries enrolled with about 45 PCPs who have gatekeeper responsibilities, including providing and authorizing covered primary and referral services.

The state pays capitation rates to KPS that represent 98.5 percent of the expected FFS expenditure for Medicaid beneficiaries in the two counties. Certain services such as drugs, dental care, and family planning are excluded and are paid through conventional Medicaid. Primary care physicians are paid a monthly capitation rate (less a reserve) for primary care services. Specialists and hospitals are paid directly by the KPS. However, beneficiary referral accounts are maintained, and pools of doctors (PODs) are used to pool the risk of referral care for the primary care managers. In this manner, residuals in these pooled accounts can be shared between primary care and specialist providers, making this a Type 2 program wherein primary care managers–gatekeepers have shared savings opportunities. If referral accounts are depleted, primary care managers in the PODs lose the primary care reserve-withholding. Stop-loss provisions are provided.

Research method

The University of Washington analysis employed several research instruments to conduct an independent evaluation of the Kitsap Sound Care Program. These instruments included a mail consumer survey to explore access and satisfaction; physician telephone interviews; other interviews with key individuals involved at the local level; a review of complaints and grievance records; a summary of the PRO's quality-of-care audit; and an analysis of cost and use data from MMIS claims. The analysis performed was primarily a descriptive one that provided an operational picture and some intercounty (Kitsap versus Mason) contrasts. The principal comparison performed in the cost and use analysis was contrasting the Sound Care enrollees to the statewide per capita cost and use rates of the nonmanaged Medicaid program. No other adjustments were made in this contrast.

The consumer survey had a response rate of approximately 55 percent, making it representative of about 15 percent of enrollees. Its questions focused on availability and accessibility of services, satisfaction, enrollment, changes in enrollments, and general understanding of the requirement of the program. The physician survey probed experience with the program and general levels of satisfaction and concern. The review of complaint logs and grievance records focused on patterns of problems detected. The PRO has a contract to do 30 case reviews per month to assess quality of care.

The cost study reported the sum of the capitation and FFS care paid for beneficiaries in the year prior to implementation and in the year since for Kitsap, Mason, and all other counties, as well as the rates of increase observed. Use rates based on claims were reported for several categories of services including inpatient and outpatient care, physician services, and drugs. The rates shown are for regular AFDC and GA combined in the most recent period and contrasted with the statewide experience in these two categories. As noted in the report, the underreporting of capitated (primary care) services was believed to be rather extensive.

Findings

While the principal interest here is in cost and use findings, some comments on the consumer survey results are appropriate. The program has seen some attrition in provider participation that has resulted in both relatively high levels of switching primary care managers (41 percent have changed) and about a quarter of enrollees saying that their prior physician did not participate in the program. In addition, there is some evidence that enrollees might not be fully apprised of all the features of gatekeeping—including access to emergency departments and to specialists—and that this problem has been a source of some concern. Access problems appear more prominent in Mason, the more rural county, where there are only seven participating PCPs.

The remaining findings are similar to those found in most other Type 1 and Type 2 programs. Quality does not appear to have been affected adversely, though no benchmark is provided either through a comparison group or preimplementation experience. Physician satisfaction is mixed but positive on balance. Complaints and grievances support some of the consumer survey findings regarding considerable provider switching behavior and some important gaps in beneficiary knowledge or understanding of the program.

With respect to cost findings, the state achieved a 1.5 percent guarantee of savings by paying 98.5 percent of the FFS equivalent per enrollee to the HIO. Looking at monthly expenditure per enrollee, the rate in Kitsap went from $62.00 in 1985 during the year prior to implementation to $73.01 in 1988, an increase of 17.8 percent. Statewide, nonmanaged Medicaid for comparable eligibility groups increased by 35.3 percent, at about two times the rate observed in Kitsap. However, the rate of increase in Mason was 52.5 percent over the same period. This increase appears to be due in part to the fact that the rate paid in Mason was the same (except for demographic differences) as in Kitsap. Since Mason is more rural than Kitsap, the preprogram expenditure level was lower. In effect, this finding indicates that Mason providers experienced substantial increases in their compensation.

The utilization analysis done for six months in 1988 (prior years had no statewide contrast data) showed that inpatient admissions in the two counties were nearly identical to the state average. Days per thousand were 10 percent lower in Kitsap and 30 percent lower in Mason, reflecting shorter LOSs. However, these figures were unadjusted for population differences. Outpatient visits (including emergency department) were considerably lower in both counties, but again, as in nonurban counties, reliance on the emergency department was typically much lower to begin with and cannot, with these data, be solely attributed to the primary care manager intervention. Physician visits were drastically lower in the two counties, but this figure lacks credibility because of obviously substantial underreporting of capitated primary care. Prescription use (uncapitated and capitated) was lower in both Kitsap (2.57) and Mason (2.52) than the statewide six-month average of 2.96.

Assessment

The introduction of this primary care manager intervention into a nonurban area using a physician service bureau as an HIO is a novel and interesting approach to extending Medicaid managed care. The Kitsap program has demonstrated feasibility and durability. The evaluation of the program reviewed offers a relatively comprehensive descriptive portrait after more than two years of operation. The evaluation was successful in many respects and detected some important strengths and weaknesses, particularly regarding operational issues.

The principal limitation of the study in terms of assessing cost and use effects was the absence of a comparison group of equivalent beneficiaries or similar counties whose experience would provide a critical frame of reference. The comparison to "all nonmanaged care beneficiaries" without any person-level adjustments is of limited usefulness. Particularly important would be the urban-versus-rural differences that would be expected to be manifested in such areas as outpatient care and emergency department use. Thus, the lower levels noted in Kitsap and Mason probably are not attributable to the primary care gatekeeper program. The other serious limitation is that the reporting of encounters by capitated providers was not rigorously monitored; thus, these data are unreliable. There is some evidence that this problem is improving, as physician visit counts have increased over time; but they are still less than one-third of the expected rates.

Washington Voluntary HMO Enrollment in Group Health Cooperative

Information sources

The source of information for this assessment was a study conducted under an NCHSR/AHCPR grant with Thomas Bice as Principal Investigator.*

Program description

The State of Washington has permitted Medicaid beneficiaries to enroll in HMOs since 1972. In the Puget Sound area, a small number of beneficiaries have enrolled in the Group Health Cooperative (GHC), a large and mature staff-model HMO with over 300,000 members. Medicaid beneficiaries in the Seattle area may choose to enroll with GHC. The plan is paid a capitation rate set at a discount from the FFS equivalent rate. During the study period for this analysis, 1984–1985, AFDC enrollment numbered approximately 5,000.

As a voluntary HMO enrollment program (Type 3) with a small enrollment in but a single HMO, this site ordinarily would not be of sufficient interest to include in the evaluation. However, as described below, the Bice study is highly informative with respect to the selection dynamics and the experience of pregnant beneficiaries. In addition, its use of both FFS Medicaid and non-Medicaid GHC enrollees as

* K. Wintringham and T. Bice, "Effects of Turnover on Use of Services by Medicaid Beneficiaries in a Health Maintenance Organization," *The Group Health Journal* 6, no. 1 (1985): 12–18.

comparison groups distinguishes it from most other analyses in terms of its thoroughness.

Research method

The focus of the Bice study was to examine the experience of Medicaid beneficiaries who had voluntarily enrolled in a well-established HMO and to contrast that experience with similar comparison groups composed of FFS Medicaid and non-Medicaid GHC members. The analysis examined utilization experience for each group, including ambulatory and inpatient use. It also reported cost per person for each category of use. The data source for this information was Medicaid claims for FFS beneficiaries and GHC encounter records with Medicaid data used to produce FFS expenditure data.

In addition to the general cost and use analysis, the study also focused specifically on the experience of prenatal care and delivery-related care. Furthermore, the evaluation addressed the extent to which enrollment in the HMO was subject to enrollment and disenrollment bias. Of special interest was how persons choosing to enroll might have pre- and postenrollment experiences that were different from the experiences of those who did not enroll. A key implication of this analysis was whether HMOs were experiencing adverse selection because of persons who chose to join having higher-than-expected use.

The selection of stratified random samples obviated the need for multivariate analyses to conduct the statistical tests of differences. Results were presented by age groups to examine whether patterns were similar among adults and children and within age segments in each group.

Findings

The final project report contains one of the most comprehensive literature reviews published on HMO experience, especially for Medicaid beneficiaries. It also presents a full and searching discussion of selection bias and its constituent literature. The evaluators did, however, limit the focus primarily to HMO enrollment experience rather than to the other models of Medicaid primary care case management.

The findings for ambulatory (outpatient) visits indicated that GHC Medicaid enrollees had significantly more visits (6.3) than non-Medicaid GHC members (4.8), but significantly fewer than FFS beneficiaries (7.4). Notably the pattern was more pronounced for women of childbearing age. With respect to type of provider, both GHC groups had a much higher proportion of their visits with primary care providers (approximately 70 percent) versus the FFS group, which had 47 percent of visits to PCPs. Some of this difference was due to higher outpatient department use for FFS persons, but specialty contacts were virtually twice as high for the FFS group.

Inpatient admissions were highest for the GHC Medicaid population (269 per 1,000) than for either the FFS (213) or the GHC general (180) populations. This difference was due to higher medical-surgical admissions in this group rather than to pregnancy, because neither of the other two groups had a higher proportion of pregnancy-related admissions. Inpatient days were lowest in the GHC general group (776) and highest in GHC Medicaid (1,434), suggesting relatively short LOSs in the former group, most of whose admissions were pregnancy related.

Total costs were highest for GHC Medicaid ($1,441) and lowest for GHC general ($821). The major source of this difference was the group of women aged 30 to 45, for whom GHC Medicaid costs were nearly three times those of general GHC members ($2,767 versus $977). Because the values to impute costs were applied to relative value units, these differences were not due to differences in costs of production (i.e., sites of services). A related analysis suggests that GHC Medicaid beneficiaries had slightly higher costs than did regular FFS beneficiaries. The authors noted that given this difference and the fact that HMO capitation rates were based on expected FFS, the HMO probably was being underpaid. In other words, although costs were higher to serve this population, the state saved money due to the enrollment of these beneficiaries in GHC.

The other analyses conducted as part of this study can be briefly summarized as follows. There appeared to have been substantial start-up costs for new Medicaid enrollees perhaps due to previously unmet needs. Although this demand leveled off, this population had a relatively short period of enrollment, approximately two years. The net effect of this short enrollment was that the level of capitation payments did not necessarily catch up with high startup use before the beneficiary disenrolled. This finding was interpreted as a disincentive to HMOs to enroll Medicaid eligibles. An analysis of enrollment and disenrollment selectivity found no evidence of use being different before or after beneficiaries joined the HMO. The analysis of outpatient care of pregnant women suggested that GHC Medicaid enrollees had use very similar to that for GHC general members. However, both groups received care that was much closer to the recommended levels observed in the FFS Medicaid group.

Assessment

Although this was a narrowly focused study of a relatively small population, it was carefully and thoroughly crafted and carried out. It is especially useful because it provides one of the most searching examinations of selectivity effects as well as startup patterns that have great significance for the viability of the HMO enrollment strategy for Medicaid. However, with only 4,500 enrollees, this is among the smallest programs examined in this evaluation.

The level of detail provided on patterns of ambulatory use is rather limited and obscures some important effects—such as emergency department use—that probably were observed. No information is presented on ancillary or prescription use, either. However, use of encounter data for a well-established HMO and the imputing of FFS equivalent payment information to relative value units of service makes the data on cost and use more credible than observed in most HMO enrollment evaluations. Conversely, the fact that the analysis applied only to one HMO, GHC, clearly restricts the generalizability of the findings. In sum, this study makes a substantial contribution in terms of some of its specific findings but is limited in its usefulness in assessing on a broader basis the impact of a major initiative of HMO Medicaid enrollment.

Wisconsin Health Maintenance Organization Program

Information sources

The program assessment is based on the state's fourth waiver renewal application and its appended internal assessment, dated March 1990.*

Program description

The state of Wisconsin initiated a mandatory HMO enrollment program in 1984 in two urban counties, Milwaukee and Dane (Madison). Although the program later expanded to Eau Claire in 1986, consolidation and dropouts in the HMO market made it impossible for the state to maintain a mandatory program in any area but Milwaukee. In February 1990, the enrollment in Milwaukee was 111,000 AFDC beneficiaries in nine HMOs. The intervention (in Milwaukee) is a mandatory enrollment program with PHPs that receive capitation for virtually the full scope of Medicaid-covered services (including dental) and that negotiate all rates with the subcontracting providers (Type 3).

The switch from mandatory to voluntary status (except in Milwaukee) introduces confounding problems that suggest that program effects are most appropriately examined in Milwaukee. However, as discussed below, because the Milwaukee area is much larger and more urbanized than the remainder of the state, analytical and operational issues are raised that need to be carefully considered when implications of the findings are assessed.

Research method

The impact analysis on cost and use focused on the covered (AFDC) beneficiaries in the counties in which the program was implemented. Because the program model entailed HMO enrollment and the HMOs were required to provide enrollees with a specifically identified PCP-gatekeeper, it is not possible to disentangle gatekeeper effects from prepayment effects. In addition, the analysis did not examine use and cost experience by specific plan, which would enable one to assess whether plan design (e.g., IPA, group) was associated with performance differences.

The basic analytical approach used was a before and after nonequivalent comparison trend analysis. A block of eight counties—asserted to be similar to the intervention counties—was selected to track the rate of change in cost and use between 1983 (preprogram) and 1989 and to compare to the rate of change in the HMO enrollment counties. In effect, this model contrasts FFS payment and use experience to capitation payment rate and use experience. The differences noted between actual and expected experience (based on comparison experience) was

---

* T. Tyson, "An Evaluation of the Medicaid HMO Program: 1987–1989" (prepared for the Evaluation Section, Office of Policy and Budget, Wisconsin Department of Health and Human Services, Madison, WI, 1989).

taken to be the program impact. Measures used in the analysis included inpatient admissions, days, average length of stay (ALOS), physician visits, emergency department visits, and prescriptions, plus expenditures per person. The measures of use were intended to come from encounter data submitted by the HMOs and monitored by the state agency. However, given the data's questionable quality, the state obtained detailed data directly from the HMOs to complete the analysis reported here. It is expected that the encounter data will be source data for future analyses.

The comparison counties were selected to provide generally comparable eligible populations to the sites with HMO enrollment. This county-level matching effort was selected in lieu of individual beneficiary-level analysis and statistical control. This approach has an important limitation inasmuch as, as noted in the report, Milwaukee is not directly comparable with any other county in the state. This problem is apparent in the utilization findings, where urban-based care patterns, such as emergency department use, were markedly different from nonurban patterns. Thus, questions about the effects of the intervention and the measurement of these effects must be raised.

With respect to generalizability, it is noteworthy that virtually all program savings at least in the past two years were due to the Milwaukee experience. That the program has become voluntary in Dane County means that selection bias would need to be appraised to establish validly what the program impact is in that county. Finally, the state has introduced copayments in the FFS Medicaid program since the HMO intervention was introduced. This history effect is noted but not controlled for in the analysis. Ignoring its impact, however, would likely err on the side of conservativism since it would dampen the rate of increase in FFS and thereby reduce the apparent savings due to the HMO.

Findings

Given the nature of the comparison versus intervention contrast, the program impacts on cost were presented in terms of relative rates of increase. The pre-HMO rate of increase to 1988–1989 (two-year average used) was 30.2 percent for the comparison counties, 14.2 percent for Milwaukee, and 32.2 percent for Dane County. During this same period, inpatient use fell by 61 percent in Milwaukee with roughly half of the decline in admissions and half in ALOS. In 1988 the inpatient use rate in HMOs was 490 per 1,000 versus 838 per 1,000 in the FFS Medicaid population.

Other measures of use displayed a mixed picture. Physician visits declined by 19 percent (one full visit) in Milwaukee over the period while ancillary use increased by 7 percent. Prescription use increased by 24 percent, but emergency department visits declined by 25 percent. The problem of the comparability of Milwaukee arises when visit rates there versus in the comparison group are examined. Despite the drop in visits, the physician visit rate in Milwaukee was still one full visit higher versus the comparison group (3.4 versus 2.4). Likewise, even after a decline of 25 percent in emergency department visits, the emergency department visit rate in Milwaukee was 4.5 times that of the comparison groups (0.59 versus 0.13) suggesting that the low rate in the comparison groups could not have changed as dramatically as in Milwaukee. This finding had the effect of potentially amplifying program impacts.

HMO program savings were calculated based on projecting comparison group rates of increases on the pre-HMO base for the intervention counties and then comparing these to the capitation outlays in the HMO enrollment counties. The savings in 1988 and 1989 were approximately $15 million in each year, net of administrative costs, and were attributed almost exclusively to the Milwaukee experience. Because the state's capitation rate included a discount of 7 to 7.5 percent of expected FFS expenditures, it virtually assured itself of savings of this magnitude.

Assessment

The principal strength of this analysis is that it was based on several years of experience and thus, at least in Milwaukee, is a portrait of a relatively mature program. There are multiple measures of use that display relatively consistent and not unexpected patterns of impact. While the analysis does examine multiple counties, confounding factors make the Milwaukee analysis the most valid. The availability of preprogram data is also highly useful.

The weaknesses include the noncomparability of Milwaukee to the comparison counties. This noncomparability is not necessarily problematic in examining overall cost trends, but does raise questions about the validity and replicability of detailed findings on use. The introduction of copayments into the FFS program was not assessed here. The inadequacy of HMO encounter data raises some questions about the potential for measurement error that was not probed in the analysis.

The use of the county as the level of analysis has several limitations. It precludes controlling for individual-level differences that might have explained differences in use and cost experience. It also exacerbates the problem of noncomparability for Milwaukee versus the remainder of the state. Finally, it does not permit examining whether there was significant variation among the participating HMOs, although such an analysis would have to have controlled for differential selection patterns.

In sum, this is a useful analysis of a mandatory HMO enrollment program with several years of operating experience in a major urban setting. Its data on cost and use impacts, while lacking a legitimate contemporaneous comparison group, are based on historic trends that are well documented.

Select Bibliography: Post-OBRA Primary Care Case Management in Medicaid

Abrams, R. "HMOs and Medicaid: Issues and Prospects." In *1986 Group Health Institute Proceedings—New Health Care Systems: HMOs and Beyond,* 37–48. Washington, DC: Group Health Association of America, 1986.

Anderson, J. "Arizona Health Care Cost Containment System." *Journal of the Florida Medical Association* 74, no. 2 (1987): 106–9.

Anderson, M., and P. Fox. "Lessons Learned from Medicaid Managed Care Approaches." *Health Affairs* 6, no. 1 (1987): 71–86.

Ashcraft, M., and S. Berki. "Health Maintenance Organizations as Medicaid Providers." *Annals of the American Academy of Political and Social Science* 468 (1983): 122–31.

Aved, B. "The Monterey County Health Initiative: A Post-Mortem Analysis of a California Demonstration Project." *Medical Care* 25, no. 1 (1987): 35–45.

Babbitt, B., and J. Rose. "Building a Better Mousetrap: Health Care Reform and the Arizona Program." *Yale Journal on Regulation* 3, no. 2 (1986): 243–82.

Babigian, H., and P. Marshall. "Rochester: A Comprehensive Capitation Experiment." *New Directions for Mental Health Services* 43 (1989): 43–54.

Batton, H., and J. Prottas. "The Complexities of Managed Care: Operating a Voluntary System." *Journal of Health Politics, Policy and Law* 2 (1987): 253–69.

Berenson, R. "A Physician's Perspective on Case Management." *Business and Health* 2 (1985): 21–24.

Bice, T. W. "Medicaid and Health Maintenance Organizations: A Review of Selectivity in Enrollment and Disenrollment." In *HMOs and Medicaid: New Initiatives and Challenges.* Washington, DC: Group Health Association of America, 1986.

Bonham, G., S. Barber, and M. Gerald. "Use of Health Care Before and During Citicare." *Medical Care* 25, no. 2 (1987): 111–19.

Bovbjerg, R., and J. Holahan. *Medicaid in the Reagan Era: Federal Policy and State Choices.* Washington, DC: Urban Institute Press, 1983.

Brecher, C. "Medicaid Comes to Arizona: A First-Year Report on AHCCCS." *Journal of Health Politics, Policy and Law* 9, no. 3 (1984): 411–25.

Buchanan, J., A. Leibowitz, J. Keesey, J. Mann, and C. Damberg. *Cost and Use of Capitated Medical Services: Evaluation of the Program for Prepaid Managed Health Care.* RAND/UCLA/Harvard Center for Health Care Financing Policy Research. Santa Monica, CA: RAND Corporation, 1992.

Burke, M. "HHS Seeks to Up Managed Care for Medicaid." *Hospitals* 64, no. 3 (1990): 70–72.

Camille, M. "State-Local Perspectives: Medicaid and HMOs: Beyond Fee for Service." *New England Journal of Human Services* 6, no. 1 (1986): 32–33.

Carter, R. "Privatization of Medicaid." *New England Journal of Human Services* 5, no. 3 (1985): 39–40.

Christianson, J. B. "Capitation of Mental Health Care in Public Programs." *Advances in Health Economics and Health Services Research* 10 (1989): 281–311.

———. "Competitive Bidding: The Challenge for Health Care Managers." *Health Care Management Review* 10, no. 2 (1985): 39–53.

———. "Provider Participation in Competitive Bidding for Indigent Patients: A Conceptual Framework and Application to the Arizona Experiment." *Inquiry* 21 (1984): 161–77.

Christianson, J. B., B. Kirkman-Liff, T. Guffey, and J. Beeler. "Nonprofit Hospitals in a Competitive Environment: Behavior in the Arizona Indigent Care Experiment." *Hospital & Health Services Administration* 32, no. 4 (1987): 475–91.

Christianson, J. B., D. G. Hillman, and R. R. Smith. "The Arizona Experiment: Competitive Bidding for Indigent Medical Care." *Health Affairs* 2 (Fall 1983): 87–103.

Christianson, J. B., and K. Smith. "Options in the Design of Competitive-Bidding Processes for Indigent Medical Care." *Contemporary Policy Issues* 3 (Winter 1984/1985): 55–68.

Christianson, J. B., N. Lurie, M. Finch, and I. Moscovice. "Mainstreaming the Mentally Ill in HMOs." In *Paying for Services: Promises and Pitfalls of Capitation,* eds. D. Mechanic and L. H. Aiken, 19–28. San Francisco: Jossey-Bass, 1989.

Christianson, J. B., R. R. Smith, and D. G. Hillman. "A Comparison of Existing Alternative Competitive Bidding Systems for Indigent Medical Care." *Social Science and Medicine* 18, no. 7 (1984): 599–604.

Cocco, A. "Gatekeeper." *Maryland Medical Journal* 35, no. 4 (1986): 273–76.

Curtis, R. "The Role of State Government in Assuring Access to Care." *Inquiry* 23, no. 3 (1986): 277–85.

Curtis, R., and J. Luehrs. "Statewide Initiatives Prompt Medicaid Recipients to Enroll in HMOs." *Business and Health* 3, no. 4 (1986): 55.

DesHarnais, S. "Enrollment in and Disenrollment from Health Maintenance Organizations by Medicaid Recipients." *Health Care Financing Review* 6, no. 3 (1985): 39–50.

DuVal, M. K. "AHCCCS: A Remarkable Success?" Letter. *Health Affairs* 5, no. 2 (1986): 156–57.

England, W. "Setting Health Maintenance Organization Capitation Rates for Medicaid in Wisconsin." *Health Care Financing Review* 7, no. 4 (1986): 67–73.

Firshein, J. "Medicaid HMO Plans to Tackle Quality Questions." *Hospitals* 60, no. 6 (1986): 76–78.

Freeman, H. E., and B. L. Kirkman-Liff. "Health Care Under AHCCCS: An Examination of Arizona's Alternative to Medicaid." *Health Services Research* 20, no. 3 (1985): 245–66.

Freund, D. A. "Competitive Health Plans and Alternative Payment Arrangements for Physicians in the U.S.: Public Sector Examples." *Health Policy* 7 (1987): 163–73.

———. "Has Public Sector Contracting with Health Maintenance Organizations in the United States Saved Money?" In *Economics in Health 1990: Proceedings of the 12th Australian Conference of Health Economists,* ed. C. Selby-Smith. Clayton, VIC: Monash University, Australian Health Economics Group, 1991.

———. "The Introduction of Competition Through Alternative Delivery Systems in the Public Sector." In *Proceedings of the Institute on Critical Issues in Health Insurance Laboratory Practice,* ed. E. Schoenfeld. Wilmington, DE: DuPont Co, 1985.

———. *Medicaid Reform: Four Studies of Case Management.* Washington, DC: American Enterprise Institute, 1984.

———. "The Private Delivery of Medicaid Services." Reprinted from the *Journal of Ambulatory Care Management* in *Alternative Delivery Systems,* eds. N. Goldfeld and S. Goldsmith. Rockville, MD: Aspen Publishers, Inc., 1987.

———. "The Private Delivery of Medicaid Services: Lessons for Administrators, Providers and Policymakers." *Journal of Ambulatory Care Management* 9, no. 2 (1986): 54–65.

Freund, D., and E. Neuschler. "Overview of Medicaid Capitation and Case Management Initiatives." *Health Care Financing Review* (1986 Annual Supplement): 21–30.

Freund, D., G. Ginsberg, L. Corder, L. Rossiter, F. Bryan, and R. Hurley. "Utilization Experiences of Medicaid Beneficiaries Enrolled in Capitated Arrangements." In *Quality Health Care in a Dynamic Era,* 212–21. Washington, DC: Group Health Association of America, 1988.

Freund, D., L. Rossiter, P. Fox, J. Meyer, R. Hurley, T. Carey, and J. Paul. "Evaluation of the Medicaid Competition Demonstrations." *Health Care Financing Review* 11, no. 2 (1989): 81–97.

Freund, D., L. Rossiter, P. Fox, L. Heinen, J. Meyer, R. Hurley, T. Carey, and J. Paul. *Integrative Final Report: Nationwide Medicaid Competition Demonstration.* HCFA Contract No. 500-83-0500. Research Triangle Park, NC: Research Triangle Institute, 1988.

Freund, D. and R. Hurley. "Managed Care in Medicaid: Selected Issues in Program Origins, Design, and Research." *Annual Review of Public Health* 8 (1987): 137–63.

Freund, D., R. Hurley, J. Paul, and C. Grubb. "Interim Findings from the Medicaid Competition Demonstrations." In *Advances in Health Economics and Health Services Research,* Vol. 10, *Risk-Based Payments Under Public Programs,* eds. R. M. Scheffler and L. F. Rossiter, 153–81. Greenwich, CT: JAI Press, Inc., 1989.

Freund, D., R. Hurley, K. Adamache, and J. Mauskopf. "The Performance of Urban and Public Hospitals and Neighborhood Health Care Centers Under Medicaid Capitated Programs." *Hospital & Health Services Administration* 35, no. 4 (1990): 525–46.

Fuller, N., and K. Koziol. "Medicaid Utilization in a Prepaid Group Practice Health Plan." *Medical Care* 15, no. 9 (1977): 705–37.

Galblum, T. K., and S. Trieger. "Demonstrations of Alternative Delivery Systems Under Medicare and Medicaid." *Health Care Financing Review* 3, no. 3 (1982): 1–12.

Garfinkel, S., W. Zelman, F. Bryan, and D. Freund. *Financial Problems Contributing to the Insolvency of the Monterey Health Initiative.* HCFA Contract No. 500-83-0050. Research Triangle Park, NC: Research Triangle Institute, 1985.

Gibson, R. "Quiet Revolutions in Medicaid." In *Market Reforms in Health Care: Current Issues, New Directions, Strategic Decisions,* ed. J. A. Meyer, 25–102. Washington, DC: American Enterprise Institute for Public Policy Research, 1983.

Gibson, R., and J. Reiss. "Health Care Delivery and Financing: Competition, Regulation, and Incentives." In *Market Reforms in Health Care: Current Issues, New Directions, Strategic Decisions,* ed. J. A. Meyer, 243–68. Washington, DC: American Enterprise Institute for Public Policy Research, 1983.

Goldfarb, N., A. Hillman, J. Eisenberg, M. Kelley, A. Cohen, and M. Dellheim. "Impact of a Mandatory Medicaid Case Management Program on Prenatal and Birth Outcomes: A Retrospective Analysis." *Medical Care* 29, no. 1 (1991): 64–71.

Gordon, T., C. Angelis, and R. Peterson. "Capitation Reimbursement for Pediatric Primary Care." *Pediatrics* 77, no. 1 (1986): 29–34.

Hadley, T., and R. Glover. "Philadelphia: Using Medicaid as a Basis for Capitation." *New Directions for Mental Health Services* 43 (1989): 65–76.

Halfon, N., and P. Newacheck. "Capitation in California—An Analysis of At-Risk Financing of Medicaid Services." *Western Journal of Medicine* 145, no. 2 (1986): 258–62.

Hillman, D. G., and J. B. Christianson. "Competitive Bidding as a Cost-Containment Strategy for Indigent Medical Care: The Implementation Experience in Arizona." *Journal of Health Politics, Policy and Law* 9, no. 3 (1984): 427–51.

Hohlen, M., L. Manheim, G. Fleming, S. Davidson, B. Yudkowsky, S. Wermer, and G. Wheatley. "Access to Office-Based Physicians Under Capitation Reimbursement and Medicaid Case Management: Findings from the Children's Medicaid Program." *Medical Care* 28, no. 1 (1990): 59–68.

Hurley, R. E. "Overview of Year Two Case Studies." In *Nationwide Evaluation of Medicaid Competition Demonstrations,* 1–74. HCFA Extramural Report No. 03236. Baltimore, MD: Health Care Financing Administration, 1986.

———. "Status of the Medicaid Competition Demonstrations." *Health Care Financing* 8, no. 2 (1986): 65–75.

———. "Toward a Behavioral Model of the Physician as Case Manager." *Social Science and Medicine* 23, no. 1 (1986): 75–82.

Hurley, R. E., and D. Freund. "Determinants of Provider Selection or Assignment in a Mandatory Case Management Program and Their Implications for Utilization." *Inquiry* 25, no. 3 (1988): 402–10.

———. "A Typology of Medicaid Managed Care." *Medical Care* 26, no. 8 (1988): 764–73.

———. "Utilization Management-Perspectives from the Medicaid Program." Paper commissioned for the Committee on Utilization Management by Third Parties, Institute of Medicine, National Academy of Sciences. Washington, DC: Institute of Medicine, 1988.

Hurley, R. E., D. Freund, and B. Gage. "Gatekeeper Effects on Patterns of Physician Use." *Journal of Family Practice* 32, no. 2 (1991): 167–74.

Hurley, R. E., D. Freund, and D. Taylor. "Emergency Room Use and Primary Care Case Management: Evidence from Four Medicaid Demonstration Programs." *American Journal of Public Health* 79, no. 7 (1989): 843–46.

———. "Gatekeeping the Emergency Room: Impact of a Medicaid Primary Care Case Management Program." *Health Care Management Review* 14, no. 2 (1989): 63–71.

Hurley, R. E., J. Paul, and D. Freund. "Going into Gatekeeping: An Empirical Assessment." *Quality Review Bulletin* 15, no. 10 (1989): 306–14.

Hurley, R. E., and M. Fennell. "Managed Care Systems as Governance Structures: A Transaction Cost Interpretation." In *Innovations in Health Care Delivery: Insights for Organizational Theory,* ed. S. Mick, 241–68. San Francisco, CA: Jossey-Bass, 1990.

Iglehart, J. "Medicaid Turns to Prepaid Managed Care." *New England Journal of Medicine* 308, no. 16 (1983): 976–80.

Iglehart, J., and J. White. "Experiments with Medicaid: Cost Containment Versus Access." *Health Progress* 68, no. 7 (1987): 26–29.

Kenkel, P. "Medicaid HMOs Struggle for Viability: Federal Plan Aims to Ease the Burden." *Modern Healthcare* 20, no. 16 (1990): 32.

Kirkman-Liff, B. "Competition in Health Care and the Rural Poor: An Assessment from Arizona's Competitive Medicaid Experiment." *Journal of Rural Health* 2, no. 1 (1986): 23–38.

Kirkman-Liff, B., F. G. Williams, and L. A. Wilson. "Medicaid and Capitated Contracting: The Arizona Experience." *New England Journal of Human Services* 5, no. 3 (1985): 30–36.

Kirkman-Liff, B., J. B. Christianson, and D. G. Hillman. "An Analysis of Competitive Bidding by Providers for Indigent Medical Care Contracts." *Health Services Research* 20, no. 5 (1985): 549–77.

Kirkman-Liff, B., J. B. Christianson, and T. Kirkman-Liff. "The Evolution of Arizona's Indigent Care System." *Health Affairs* 6, no. 4 (1987): 46–58.

Kleinman, J., M. Gold, and D. Makuc. "Use of Ambulatory Care Medical Care by the Poor." *Medical Care* 19, no. 10 (1981): 1011–29.

Krasner, W. "New Directions in Medicare and Medicaid Managed Care." *Medical Staff Counselor* 2, no. 4 (1988): 23–29.

Langwell, K. "Structure and Performance of Health Maintenance Organizations: A Review." *Health Care Financing Review* 12, no. 1 (1990): 71–79.

Levy, A. A., J. E. Greenidge, and N. C. Monti. "Successful Outreach and Market Strategies for Medicaid Subscribers in a Large, Urban HMO." In *Proceedings of the 30th Annual Group Health Institute—Skills Development for the HMO*

Managers of the 1980s. Washington, DC: Group Health Association of America, 1980.

Levy, M. "Containing Medicaid Costs and Improving Services Through Primary Care Networks: The Kansas Experience." *New England Journal of Human Services* 5, no. 3 (1985): 26–29.

Long, S., and R. Settle. "An Evaluation of Utah's Primary Care Case Management Program for Medicaid Recipients."*Medical Care* 26, no. 11 (1988): 1021–32.

Mauch, D. "Rhode Island: An Early Effort at Managed Care." *New Directions for Mental Health Services* 43 (1989): 55–64.

McCall, N., D. Henton, M. Crane, S. Haber, D. Freund, and W. Wrightson. "Evaluation of the Arizona Health Care Cost Containment System (AHCCCS): The First Eighteen Months." *Health Care Financing Review* 7, no. 2 (1985): 77–88.

McCall, N., D. Henton, S. Haber, L. Paringer, M. Crane, W. Wrightson, and D. Freund. "Evaluation of Arizona Health Care Cost Containment System (AHCCCS)." *Health Care Financing Review* 9, no. 2 (1987): 79–89.

McCombs, J. S., and J. B. Christianson. "Applying Competitive Bidding to Health Care." *Journal of Health Politics, Policy and Law* 12, no. 4 (1987): 703–22.

Merrill, J. "Defining Case Management." *Business and Health* 2, no. 8 (1985): 5–9.

Moscovice, I., M. Finch, and N. Lurie. "Minnesota: Plan Choices by the Mentally Ill in Medicaid Prepaid Health Plans." *Advances in Health Economics and Health Services Research* 10 (1989): 265–78.

Mulcahy, E. "New HMOs for Medicaid Patients Expected to Harm EDs Financially." *Emergency Department News* 6, no. 10 (1984): 1–28.

National Governors' Association. *Prepaid and Managed Care Under Medicaid.* Washington, DC: The Association, 1985.

Oberg, C. "Medicaid and Managed Healthcare: Enrollment in HMOs and Other Alternative Health Systems." *GHAA Journal* 8, no. 1 (1987): 49–62.

Oberg, C., and C. Polich. *1987 Medicaid and HMO Data Book: The Expansion of Capitated Managed Care Systems.* Excelsior, MN: InterStudy, 1988.

Orient, J. E. "The Arizona Health Care Cost Containment System: A Prepayment Model for a National Health Service?" *Western Journal of Medicine* 145, no. 1 (1986): 114–23.

Prottas, J., and E. Handler. "The Complexities of Managed Care: Operating a Voluntary System." *Journal of Health Care Politics, Policy and Law* 12, no. 2 (1987): 253–69.

Riley, P., A. Coburn, and E. Kilbreth. *Medicaid Managed Care: The State of the Art—A Guide for States.* Portland, ME: National Academy for State Health Policy and the Edmund S. Muskie Institute of Public Affairs, University of Southern Maine, 1990.

Rosenbaum, S., D. Hughes, F. Butler, and D. Havard. "Incantations in the Dark: Medicaid, Managed Care, and Maternity Care." *Milbank Memorial Fund Quarterly* 66, no. 1 (1988): 661–93.

Rosenblatt, R. "Medicaid Primary Care Case Management: The Doctor-Patient Relationship and the Politics of Privatization." *Case Western Reserve University Law Review* 36 (1986): 915–68.

Rossiter, L., D. Freund, R. Hurley, and M. Jurgenson. "Medicaid Case Management Programs: What Are the Cost Impacts and Implications for Providers?" *Health Care Management Review* (forthcoming).

Rowland, D., and B. Lyons. "Mandatory HMO Care for Milwaukee's Poor." *Health Affairs* 6, no. 1 (1987): 87–100.

Schaller, D., A. Bostrom, and J. Rafferty. "Quality of Care: Recent Experience in Arizona." *Health Care Financing Review* (1986 Annual Supplement): 65–74.

Segodnia, W. "Medicaid Capitation Rates: Methodological Shortcomings and Recommended Solutions." *Group Health Association of America Journal* 9, no. 2 (1988): 83–95.

Silverstein, G., J. K. Olsen-Garewale, and S. Yates. "AHCCCS in Rural Arizona: The Gatekeeper Role Explored." In *1986 Group Health Proceedings—New Health Care Systems: HMOs and Beyond,* 95–101. Washington, DC: Group Health Association of America, 1986.

Smith, V., and S. Hetrick. "Primary Care Case Management for Medicaid Clients: Michigan's Response." *New England Journal of Human Services* 7, no. 2 (1987): 33–34.

Spitz, B. "Medicaid Case Management: Lessons for Business." *Business and Health* 2, no. 8 (1985): 16–21.

———. "A National Survey of Medicaid Case Management Programs." *Health Affairs* 6, no. 1 (1987): 61–70.

———. "Primary Care Physicians for Medicaid Patients." *New England Journal of Human Services* 6, no. 4 (1986): 33–34.

———. "When a Solution Is Not a Solution: Medicaid and Health Maintenance Organizations." *Journal of Health Politics, Policy and Law* 3, no. 4 (1979): 497–518.

Spitz, B., and J. Abramson. "Competition, Capitation, and Case Management: Barriers to Strategic Reform." *Milbank Memorial Fund Quarterly* 65, no. 3 (1987): 348–68.

Temkin-Greener, H. "Medicaid Families Under Managed Care: Anticipated Behavior." *Medical Care* 24, no. 8 (1986): 721–32.

Temple, P. C., and S. Kron. "The Philadelphia Health Insurance Organization: The Results of Managed Health Care for 96,000 Medical Assistance Recipients." *Health Matrix* 7, no. 4 (1990): 12–20.

Traska, R. "WA Medicaid Study Challenges HMO Care Myths." *Hospitals* 61, no. 15 (1987): 42–44.

U.S. General Accounting Office. *Medicaid: Lessons Learned from Arizona's Prepaid Program.* GAO/HRD-87-14. Washington, DC: U.S. GAO, 1987.

———. *Medicaid: Oversight of Health Maintenance Organizations in the Chicago Area.* GAO/HRD-90-81. Washington, DC: U.S. GAO, 1990.

Vertrees, J., K. Manton, and K. Mitchell. "Case Mix Adjusted Analyses of Service Utilization for a Medicaid Health Insuring Organization in Philadelphia." *Medical Care* 27, no. 4 (1989): 397–411.

Vogel, R. "An Analysis of Structural Incentives in the Arizona Health Care Cost-Containment System." *Health Care Financing Review* 5, no. 4 (1984): 13–22.

Wan, T. T. H. "The Effect of Managed Care on Health Services Use by Dually Eligible Elders." *Medical Care* 27, no. 1 (1989): 983–1001.

Welch, W. P. "Giving Physicians Incentives to Contain Costs Under Medicaid," *Health Care Financing Review* 12, no. 2 (1990): 103–12.

———. "HMO Enrollment and Medicaid: Survival Analysis with a Weibull Function." *Medical Care* 26, no. 1 (1988): 48–52.

Welch, W., and M. Miller. ''Mandatory HMO Enrollment in Medicaid: The Issue of Freedom of Choice.'' *Milbank Memorial Fund Quarterly* 66, no. 4 (1988): 618–39.

Wintringham, K., and T. Bice. ''Effects of Turnover on Use of Services by Medicaid Beneficiaries in a Health Maintenance Organization.'' *The Group Health Journal* 6, no. 1 (1985): 12–18.

Index

About the Authors

Robert E. Hurley, Ph.D., is an assistant professor at the Medical College of Virginia/Virginia Commonwealth University in the Department of Health Administration. He received an M.S. degree in hospital and health services administration from Ohio State University and a Ph.D. in health policy and administration from the University of North Carolina at Chapel Hill. His teaching and research interests are in the area of managed care and organizational theory.

Deborah A. Freund, Ph.D., is a professor of health economics and associate dean in the School of Public and Environmental Affairs at Indiana University. She holds academic appointments both in the Department of Economics and in the School of Medicine. In addition, she directs the Otis Bowen Health Services Research Center at Indiana University. Dr. Freund received her M.A., M.P.H., and Ph.D. degrees in public health and economics at the University of Michigan. She has published extensively, most notably in the areas of managed care, Medicaid, and hospital length of stay. Dr. Freund has received numerous awards and currently serves on the boards of directors of the Association of University Programs in Health Administration and the Association for Health Services Research.

John E. Paul, Ph.D., is a senior research health analyst at Research Triangle Institute. He received his M.S.P.H. and his Ph.D. in health policy and administration from the School of Public Health, University of North Carolina at Chapel Hill. He has been working at Research Triangle Institute since 1983, primarily in the areas of Medicaid and Medicare organization and financing.